RECALIBRATE

RECALIBRATE

Six Secrets to Resetting Your Age

Richard Purvis

Printed in the United States of America

First Printing: 2017

Title ID: 7660196
ISBN-13: 9781978441699
ISBN-10: 197844169X
Library of Congress Control Number: 2017917928
CreateSpace Independent Publishing Platform
North Charleston, South Carolina

Dedications

*For my mother, who first exposed me to various
wellness platforms back in the 70s.*

*For my life-partner, Stephanie, who has been incredibly supportive
and encouraging throughout the process of this book.*

*And for my son, Alastair, who I am so proud of for grasping
and integrating wellness into his life so early on.*

"We are what we repeatedly do. Excellence, then, is not an act, but a habit"

~ **ARISTOTLE**

Contents

Introduction Sowing The Seeds ·xi

1 A Doctor's Discovery · 1
2 Impact of Our Lifestyles · 8
3 Nutritional Intake · 27
4 Exercise = Life Extension · 66
5 In Need of Supplements? · 95
6 Intermittent Fasting · 114
7 Weight Loss · 127
8 Healthy Gut - Healthy Brain · 134
9 Sleep · 143
10 Your Best Skin · 155
11 Connection = Happiness & Longevity? · · · · · · · · · · · · · · 172

References · 179

Introduction
Sowing The Seeds

"Let us cultivate our garden."

~ VOLTAIRE

Some people experience an awareness of their life's work at an early age. That was not exactly the case with me. I admit, even as a young boy I had a fascination with people, specifically with physical appearances and what made a person look a certain way. By the time I was nearing college, a passion that led to my career path had ignited.

I grew up in Southern California in the 60s. Perhaps my intrigue with how people look was simply a part of my environment. Some of my earliest memories involved pondering why a person looked a particular way – fat versus thin, tan versus pale, wrinkled and lined skin versus smooth skin, and squared faces versus round or oval faces etc.

At some point in my youth, I became intrigued by what caused a person to look good or bad, healthy or unhealthy, aged or youthful. I asked questions relentlessly to determine what things were healthy. "Dad, is mowing the yard really that good for me?"

His answers were somewhat predictable. "Yes, hard work is good for you Richard, it teaches you a strong work ethic, discipline, and an appreciation that nothing in life is free." Not exactly the answer my inquisitive mind wanted.

I spent my teenage summers in Alaska alternating between working on fishing boats or pumping gas and repairing tires in a gas station. I remember hoping my dad's assessment of how hard work is good for me was accurate. The summer's many long days of grueling, physical labor certainly provided the opportunity to prove his theory. I often wondered if the combination of the exertion combined with the exposure to the elements would make me look like some of the locals and I studied their deeply-lined faces and leathery skin.

During the same period of my late teens, my interest in vitamins was piqued. Suddenly, vitamin supplements were everywhere. I came home from Alaska following a summer break and found my mother deeply committed to the vitamin vogue. She had cupboards full of bottles, bags, and boxes containing an alphabet of the healthy-life transformers. Mother had converted to the Amway and Shaklee doctrine – she was a believer.

The timing for my immersion into the wondrous world of vitamins was perfect. The tenuous fear of looking like a weathered Alaskan fisherman prompted me to start going through my mother's arsenal seeking a preventative. My experimentation began with taking one of my mom's multi-vitamins. I noticed no marked change in my physical appearance until I urinated. I noticed my urine was a much darker, yellow color and it had a distinct smell. I later learned the odor was a byproduct of the concentration of B vitamins. That evidence of my body's processing served as validation. I thought to myself, *Wow, these things must work.* It was my epiphany! The consuming interest in nutritional health and the subsequent devotion to my life's work became officially galvanized.

Unfortunately, commitment to my physical health and appearance did not inspire an entirely wholesome lifestyle. In college I began to do what most students do, I partied. I thoroughly enjoyed the social participation of the party scene but, I did not like how I felt the day after drinking; dehydrated, slow, bleary, bloated, achy, and dull.

I often thought about the Alaskan fishermen's faces, and I became convinced if I continued the routine practice of partying, I would end up looking just like that – or worse. The conviction motivated me to not only participate in less partying but to continue to learn as much as I could about nutrition and health. By the time I left college, I was totally immersed in striving for a holistic well-being. I studied everything I could find and I read (1) ate, drank, and slept with the ultimate goal of my healthy lifestyle in mind. I incorporated a regimented eating, exercising, and a supplement program into my daily routine. My experience and passion led to goals that included building a reputable supplement company.

In 1986, I met a South African woman visiting the United States, and I became captivated by my first, significant, romantic relationship. She inspired me to move to her beautiful hometown of Durban, KwaZulu-Natal, and we ultimately married.

Life in South Africa provided a momentous personal awakening. The country, entrenched in the anti-apartheid revolution was considered a pariah state. Living in South Africa, I witnessed the consequences of its colonial history, the force of segregation, and the effects of the resistance that was created from it and I was captivated by it all.

I was a child of the tumultuous 1960s. It was during that period the US was forced to confront its own civil rights issues and the local and national news was filled with stories of riots, protests, and unrest. I had a smidgen of an understanding of the struggle of African citizens and felt sympathetic.

Desire to support their plight for equality prompted us to more consciously treat our African employees well. We worked to teach advanced job skills, offering advancement opportunity as the main motivating factor. One special employee and friend, Simon Mogano, started with us as a retailer stockist and worked his way up to management. He remains in contact with me to this day, after all, these many years.

I was enthralled by the euphoria of the South African people when political activist Nelson Mandela gained release from prison. I reveled in the country's jubilation and optimism in 1994 when Mandela was elected South Africa's first black president.

The 19 years I spent in South Africa represented as much a time of transformation for me individually as it did for the country. It was a period of major conversion, and it epitomized an era of tremendous hope. Watching a man like Nelson Mandela emerge from prison and become President of this bitter, segregated county produced an indelible impact. I recall thinking, *how can this man not seek revenge for what the Afrikaners did to him?* He was imprisoned, and subjected to hard labor for 27 years because of his political beliefs! When finally freed, his motivating desire was to repair his broken country. To this day, Mandela's demonstration of courage and selflessness remains a most remarkable, personal inspiration.

Within a few years of my arrival in South Africa, I managed to obtain a pivotal goal and I started a nutritional supplement company. I named the organization *Nutrimax*.

Persistent competitive research and due diligence during the initial business development phase revealed many competitors were introducing bogus supplements to the marketplace. Standard regulations for supplements in those early days were lax, product labels bore inaccurate ingredient lists, and compounds were packaged and sold in poor quality and synthesized forms. A significant problem with misnaming certain additives, especially those synthesized in labs, exists because certain formulations are simply not absorbable. Ultimately, the critical elements are eliminated from the body serving no nutritional benefit whatsoever, and possibly even doing a bit of harm if over used as that could create toxicity.

Our founding philosophy was to ensure that every ingredient we used was 'food state' meaning the molecular structure was similar to the values of nutrients found in whole foods and with similar bioavailability. The 'purity concept' was unique at the time but I felt it essential to protect the integrity of the products, their efficacy, and ultimately our brand. It is the corporate standard my companies maintain to this day.

Although supplements were not a new concept in South Africa during the late 1980s and early 1990s, the types of products we were producing were unique and innovative. We concentrated on formulating the best quality products that yielded 'food state' nutrient values, high-bioavailability, maximum efficacy, and line items that no other company was offering at the time. The knowledge base and prior industry experience I offered made a huge difference in the company's ability to create and articulate a resonating message to our consumers. We initially focused on sports nutrition and gradually moved into more general wellness and finally into anti-aging products.

The same industry experience served me well in a very personal capacity as well. While visiting a game reserve in the African bushveld, a mosquito carrying encephalitis infected me with the deadly virus. Within a few days of the insect's bite I suffered acute complications from the disease including a raging fever and swelling in my brain.

The treating doctors' efforts did little to effectively control the symptoms of the virus. My physicians expressed concern with the severity of the brain swelling. They recommended a ventriculostomy. A tube would be inserted and the fluid building in my brain drained if the swelling continued to worsen. They advised if left untreated, I could suffer permanent brain damage.

None of the medical treatments presented were attractive. I decided to try something on my own and immediately started taking elevated doses of high potency DHA/EPA fish oil in an effort to reduce inflammation and protect my brain. I added phosphatidylserine, phosphatidylcholine, and Vitamin D for further protection, and I started a cleansing diet of high nutrient value, dark, richly colored vegetables and berries to help boost my immune system and flush out the toxins. Within a few days of my nutritional intervention, the swelling in my brain reversed and soon after that, all other symptoms of the encephalitis disappeared. My doctors evaluated a battery of subsequent tests and concluded that I had indeed rid myself of the virus as well as escaped brain damage.

I am not recommending anyone should ever attempt an extreme experiment such as this. My personal experience is NOT a claim to a cure for severe, complicated medical conditions. I am merely pointing out the knowledge that I gained over years of experience helped me make an educated decision about my treatment options. I was willing to become my own guinea pig. Medically my somewhat miraculous recovery remains open for debate. It may or may not be due to my personal, nutritional intervention. I choose to believe it did and the efficacy of the treatment probably saved me from suffering permanent damage.

After 15 years I moved away from the supplement business, and I now concentrate my efforts in the wellness and anti-aging industry, focusing on lifestyle choices that include what we put into our mouths, onto our skin, and exercise. Throughout my journey, I've remained committed to researching everything related to wellness available to me. I have personally tried and tested numerous supplements, eating plans, exercise routines, and every topical application imaginable. **Recalibrate** represents a compilation of what I have found makes the biggest individual difference.

I detail the most dependable, most efficacious ways of optimizing the anti-aging process. I evaluate methods to not only look and feel younger, but how to create excellent holistic health – for life.

People often ask, "What got you into this industry?" My answer is never a simple one. Many factors contributed to my vision, my passion, and to my career. When I consider the chronological order, it's as if each life experience cemented an integral piece of the path for me.

Whether by happenchance, environment, or intuition, an early curiosity possessed me as to why something may or may not be "good" for me. I was intrigued about why some people looked more aged and weathered than others. I didn't always get it right, and I made some bad decisions along the way, but taking care of my body was always of critical importance to me.

In more recent years, I became particularly motivated by the aspiration to share what I have learned on my journey. It is the objective to help others reach their personal goals through my enlightenment that inspired me to write **Recalibrate.**

I find most people establish personal health and wellness goals that are absolutely attainable, yet they consistently fail. The paradigm is troubling. I believe the reason for most failure is often the result of simply looking in the wrong places for direction and exercising the wrong options to achieve success.

Many companies are only interested in selling products for monetary gain. They distribute vague and often misleading product information to achieve their objective. Commercial food manufacturers have little regard for the nutritional value of their goods; unfortunately, some supplement companies are just as bad. A lot of books are written under the guise of providing quality information from an "expert's view" of a subject and, in reality, they are nothing more than propaganda to market at best, marginal products. It's all about profitability!

Here I must offer a full disclosure; I do own a skin care company and am part owner in a nutritional snack bar business. My objective for writing this book however, is not about selling my products. My absolute intent is to educate consumers about methods to achieve better overall health and wellness without any hidden agendas.

My motivation goes well beyond how to improve one's appearance. The risk of developing a chronic illness increases exponentially with each birthday. Lifestyle choices we make accelerate the aging process and this makes us more susceptible to certain diseases such as diabetes, obesity, hypertension, cancer, heart disease, arthritis, and the dreaded Alzheimer's. What are we doing to ourselves to trigger all these diseases? More importantly, what are we not doing to prevent them and what can we do at any stage of life to fend them off?

What is the quality of a life that is dependent on the daily pill for blood pressure, another for cholesterol, another for arthritis, and so on? Sure, doctors can extend a physical existence with a plethora of medications, but it is how you choose to spend the later stage of life – the "golden years" – that goes beyond just existing and should be considered now.

A dependency on drug therapy doesn't have to be your future, my friends! There are measures you can take right now to change that fate and afford the ability to live life on your terms. Practicing good health will not only provide the best opportunity to avoid the potential of 'self-induced' diseases, but it will also dramatically improve the quality of life and help you look and feel better than you have in a decade. Applying my proven techniques will facilitate a more youthful and radiant appearance as well superior overall health!

Enjoy the journey and get ready to embrace a new you!

1

A Doctor's Discovery

"If you don't like something, change it. If you can't change it, change your attitude."

~ MAYA ANGELOU

In 1999 I was well into the personal journey to improve my knowledge of nutrition and supplements and how each contributed to my overall health. I sought every resource I could find to study the principals of the subject. One day I picked up an updated edition *of Nutrition and Physical Degeneration* by Dr. Weston Price, D.D.S. The original edition of the book was practically ancient. It was first published in 1939 and Dr. Price was not a nutritionist but a dentist!

Needless to say, I was skeptical about any relevant information this documentation would provide my current studies, but I bought the book, so I had to read on. All I can say is, "WOW!" Dr. Price's exploration and research certainly opened my eyes. His moniker as the "Issac Newton of Nutrition" is certainly well deserved. I feel his findings regarding nutrition are so important that I hope to distil some of the most significant discoveries for my readers. Interestingly, I find his information in the book ever more relevant today than when I first bought it.

Dr. Weston Price was a practicing dentist in Cleveland, Ohio in the 1930s. Increasingly disturbed by the amount of tooth decay he witnessed in his patients, Price sought answers to what he perceived as something of an anomaly.

Dr. Price noticed many of his younger patients had increasingly deformed dental arches, crooked teeth, and far more cavities than similarly aged patients just a decade or so earlier. He also noticed a strong correlation between dental health and physical health (e.g. a mouth full of cavities went hand in hand with a body either full of disease, or generalized poor health and susceptibility to disease).

He deliberated as to the cause of these unexpected changes and knew that they were highly abnormal. He had heard rumors of populations untouched by western civilization where the people were virtually free of tooth problems and other diseases. Dr. Price researched these rumored communities a bit further, and as he did, his intrigue grew.

The initial findings and intrigue were enough to impel Dr. Price into what would become a series of explorations that spanned the globe for more than ten years.

The communities Dr. Price included on his radar included; remote villages in Switzerland, Gaelic communities in the Outer Hebrides, and Inuits of Alaska, the Native Americans of the Pacific Northwest and central Canada. His interest encompassed the Melanesians and Polynesians, Aborigines of Australia, the Maori of New Zealand, descendants of the ancient Chimú culture in coastal Peru, and certain tribes of Africa, including; Maasai, Kikuyu, Wakamba, Jalou, Muhima, Pygmies, Bantu, and Dinkas.

Dr. Price visited all of these communities and more with the goal of establishing what was behind their almost non-existent dental and health issues. In each location, he examined, assessed, and analyzed the people in these communities, photographing teeth, faces and other features he found interesting (he took more than 15,000 photographs), as well as recording the general health and the dietary habits of the various cultures.

In every community, of the dozens he studied, without exception, he found that tooth decay, tooth loss, dental abscesses or infections were very uncommon, typically affecting no more than one to three percent (and sometimes none) of the teeth he examined. He also noted the absence of gingivitis and periodontitis, and few to no deformed bridges, crooked or crowded teeth. Dr. Price further observed that facial structures were different with these cultures, enjoying what he called "fully formed facial and dental arches" and a lack of narrowed nasal passages as well as good physiques and seemingly high resistance to disease.

Interestingly, Dr. Price also sought out members of these cultures who recently transitioned to consuming Western foods, such as people who had started trading with Westerners visiting their lands, bartering for bread, pastries, and other sweets. In every instance, he observed an astounding increase in tooth decay, affecting 25% to 50% of teeth examined, along with gingivitis, periodontitis, tooth loss, infectious abscesses, crooked and crowded teeth, and reductions in the size of the maxillary (mid-facial) bone and mandible (jawbone).

What is even more intriguing about Dr. Price's annotations was the rarity of tooth decay and deformity in the cultures that had not partaken in the consumption of Western foods. None of these cultures practiced any dental hygiene - no toothbrushes, no toothpaste, no fluoridated water, no dental floss and no dentists or orthodontists. While Dr. Price's observations do not precisely pinpoint the nutritional distinctions between modern and traditional cultures, they nonetheless make a significant point.

The cultural diets of these societies were totally natural and unprocessed. They did not consist of white flour, added sugar, or canned foods.

They ate animals that naturally grazed on plants and grasses, organic plant foods, fish, shellfish, and sea vegetables, raw dairy products, and nuts and seeds etc.

Dr. Price noted only two cultures he encountered ate grains. A group of people in the Lotschental Valley, Switzerland whose diet primarily consisted of dairy products (raw milk, butter, cream and raw milk cheese) from cows grazing on lush alpine slopes, and rye bread (they called it roggenbrot), made from rye that they grew themselves in their fertile soils. They did eat meat occasionally, and some vegetables during their summers.

The other group, the Gaelic people of the islands of the Outer Hebrides, consumed primarily sea foods and oat foods such as porridge and oat cakes (not a bastardized Western processed food that would be full of sugar), more like a flatbread that was made of pounded and ground oats. Dr. Price noted that there were a few minor instances of very mild tooth decay in the Swiss and none noted for the Gaelic people.

Dr. Price was eager to analyze the chemical composition of the various foods these primitive cultures consumed. He was careful to obtain preserved samples of all types for his studies. After analysis of the preserved samples, Dr. Price concluded the diets of the individual, healthy cultures contained ten times the amount of fat-soluble vitamins, and at least four times the amount of calcium, other minerals, and water soluble vitamins than Western diets for that period. The concentration of fermented and raw foods (including raw animal products) consumed led Dr. Price to note the natural diets rich in enzymes enabled easier digestion and assimilation and improved the overall digestion of cooked foods.

Dr. Price's studies led him to believe all cultures had a predilection and dietary pull towards foods rich in the fat-soluble vitamins. He considered butter from pasture-fed cows rich in these vitamins as well as minerals, to be the premiere health food. Fat-soluble vitamins are found in fats of animal origin, like butter, cream, lard, and tallow, as well as in organ meats.

Dr. Price's research dispelled a common myth regarding native people's limited longevity. He took numerous photos of healthy individuals from various cultures with heads full of gray hair. While the photos did not document exactly how old the subjects were (most native tribes did not use calendars) by all appearances, each person was well past 60 years of age.

Dr. Price's comprehensive and meticulous studies concluded that tooth decay and deformed dental arches resulting in crowded, crooked teeth, were primarily the result of consumption of certain food types (such as excessive carbohydrates). These destructive foods promote specific types of bacteria, which produce acid that destroys the tooth's enamel and its underlying layer-- the dentin. It is nutritional deficiencies -- not inherited genetic defects -- that contribute to poor dental health as well as other individual physical issues.

Below is a glimpse at some of the notable differences in traditional diets and modern diets:

Traditional Diets

- Plant foods from fertile soil
- Organ meats preferred over muscle meats
- Natural animal fats
- Animals that fed on pasture such as grasses and plants - without hormones, grains, and antibiotics
- Dairy products raw and/or fermented
- Grains and legumes (if and when consumed) soaked and/or fermented
- Soy foods given long fermentation, consumed in small amounts

- Fermented vegetables
- Fermented beverages
- Unrefined salt
- Seeds
- Traditional cooking methods

Modern Diets

- Foods from depleted soil
- Primarily muscle meats, limited organ meats
- Processed vegetable oils
- Animals in confinement raised on grain, antibiotics, and hormones
- Dairy products pasteurized or ultra-pasteurized
- Grains refined, and/or extruded
- Soy foods industrially processed, consumed in large amounts
- MSG, artificial flavorings
- Refined sweeteners
- Processed, pasteurized pickles
- Refined salt
- Synthetic vitamins ingested alone or added as supplements to foods
- Microwave, Irradiation
- Hybrid seeds, GMO seeds

So, how do we correlate Dr. Price's findings nearly 100 years ago and the nutritional health crisis today? The root causes are the same; the devastating effects amplified. Individual lifestyles and poor dietary habits continually damage the body's cells. We are not only causing tooth decay and dental health problems, but major bodily deterioration is manifesting in a multitude of ways.

Dr. Price's findings and conclusions were highly illuminating and are still being debated and referenced today. *Nutrition and Physical Degeneration* is currently in its 8th edition and 23rd printing! His studies of isolated non-industrialized peoples established the parameters of human health and determined the optimum characteristics of human diets. Dr. Price's research demonstrated that humans achieve perfect physical form and optimum health generation after generation only when they consume nutrient-dense whole foods and vital fat-soluble activators found exclusively in animal fats. A foundation in 1999 was created in his honor, called The Weston A. Price Foundation. It is a nonprofit, tax-exempt charity founded to disseminate the research of the nutrition pioneer.

The Foundation (1) remains dedicated to restoring nutrient-dense foods to the human diet through education, research, and activism. It supports movements that contribute to this objective including; accurate nutrition instruction, organic and biodynamic farming, pasture-feeding of livestock, community-supported farms, honest and informative labeling, prepared parenting and nurturing therapies. Specific goals include the establishment of universal access to clean, certified raw milk and a ban on the use of soy formula for infants.

I highly recommend reading the masterpiece *Nutrition and Physical Degeneration* by Dr. Weston Price as it highlights his critical discoveries and conclusions. The book features striking photographs of robust, healthy, peoples visually illustrating the physical degeneration that occurs when human groups abandon nourishing traditional diets for nutritionally barren, modern convenience foods.

2

Impact of Our Lifestyles

"As long as a person stands in their own way, everything seems to be in their way."

~ *RALPH WALDO EMERSON*

The amount of junk food, processed food, sugar, simple carbs, and bad fats in most Western diets is creating a huge population of sick and overweight people. We are highly stressed, take too many medications, and do not get enough exercise. The combination of poor lifestyle choices not only makes way for disease and physical decay, but it also serves to age our bodies prematurely. The saddest part of the individual's demise is the FACT -- it is self-induced!

While there are many unhealthy aspects of the typical Western diet, the problems not only begin with overall poor consumer choices, but misinformation also plays a significant role in our eating behaviors. The United States Department of Agriculture (USDA) publishes flawed and misguided nutritional advice. Historically, USDA recommendations include the daily consumption of foods heavy in grains and low in healthy fats, which no doubt fuels epidemics like obesity, diabetes, and other chronic disorders. Traditionally, the USDA Food Pyramid recommended 6-11 servings of bread cereals, rice, and pasta. This 'grain group' represents the base of the food pyramid and the largest daily dietary cluster. The revised pyramid published in 2015 reduced recommended daily intake of these foods marginally to 4-8 servings.

You might ask, "Well, what is wrong with eating 6-11 or 4-8 servings of these foods?" The simple answer is to consider the design of the human body. Our bodies utilize food for energy and to store fat to use for energy at a later stage. Our ancient ancestors did not have the luxury of eating as much as they wanted anytime they wanted, like we do. They were hunter-gatherers and the ability to store fat was essential to survival when they could not find food for extended periods of time.

The modern human body processes food in much the same way. The trouble begins with the overabundant amounts of food available today, and specifically the wrong kinds of foods such as simple carbohydrates. We consume way too much food, especially foods from the base of the USDA's food pyramid, the 'grain group' foods, in shorter intervals causing our bodies to go into a perpetuating cycle of storing fat.

Our body's ability to store fat begins whenever we eat. The digestion system breaks food down into glucose, which then makes its way into the bloodstream. The introduction of glucose signals the pancreas to produce a hormone called insulin. Insulin is released by the pancreas into the bloodstream to shuttle the glucose to various cells throughout the body. From there it is used for energy or stored as fat. Insulin also signals the bodies' cells to open up and absorb the glucose.

As the glucose is slowly absorbed into cells, insulin levels drop, and the pancreas waits for us to eat food again to repeat the process. When too much food is consumed, particularly too many carbohydrates, excessive amounts of glucose is released into the bloodstream causing the pancreas to produce extra insulin to deal with it. The body must store the glucose it cannot immediately use as fat.

On the average, American adults consume more than 300 grams of carbohydrates per day. We know excessive carbohydrate consumption shoves the body into a permanent state of fat storage and it is the primary cause of obesity and many other health issues. It produces an enormous strain on the pancreas to manufacture adequate amounts of insulin. The over-taxed pancreas will ultimately break down causing severe health conditions such as Type-2 diabetes.

Another important hormone affected by this dreadful cycle is leptin, often referred to as the "satiety hormone" or the "starvation hormone." Leptin is a cell-signaling hormone vital to the regulation of appetite, food intake, energy expenditure, and body weight.

In a properly functioning body, fat cells in adipose tissue produce and release leptin, sending signals to the brain. The particular brain function affected by this process is the hypothalamus, which triggers and regulates the appetite.

The amount of leptin released to the brain is directly related to the amount of body fat a person produces. Consequently, the more body fat an individual has, the more leptin circulates in the blood. Leptin levels increase if the fat mass surges over a period and similarly, leptin levels decrease if an individual effectively reduces their fat mass.

Unfortunately, an obese individual typically produces too much leptin leading to a lack of sensitivity to the hormone. The medical condition is known as "leptin resistance." Leptin resistance results in the brain's inability to respond properly to the hormone, so the individual keeps eating because there is no signal telling them they are satiated. That obviously results in a bad situation getting worse!

Leptin and insulin are negatively influenced by similar things, and their biggest transgressors are carbohydrates. The more refined and processed the carbohydrate, the more out of whack healthy levels of leptin and insulin become. Both critical hormones act as pro-inflammatory agents as well.

INFLAMMATION - THE ROOT OF DISEASE!

When it comes to your health, inflammation is public enemy number one. Inflammation is the major contributor to virtually every identified, age-related disease.

Dr. Michael Roizen is one of America's leading experts on preventive medicine and serves as the chairman of the world-famous Cleveland Clinic's Wellness Institute. He is the author of numerous best-selling books as well as the co-founder of the successful *RealAge*. *RealAge* is a scientifically based assessment factoring in lifestyle, genetics, and medical history, that tells you how old your body thinks you are based on your health and health habits.

Roizen points to the latest research indicating inflammation as the root of nearly every medical problem regardless of severity:

> Whether you have a wrinkle in your skin caused by an inflamed artery, or a wrinkle in your heart; a heart attack, or impotence, it's really the same process, and it's all caused, or at least it starts with inflammation.

> Inflammation is the silent killer that has eluded the medical community for years. It's only recently that we've understood that it has an important or prominent role in causing diseases such as cancer, heart attacks, and strokes, or of causing the infectious diseases we now have getting out of control.

So what's causing all of the troubling inflammation? We mentioned the role insulin and leptin play in the effective functioning of the body. Consequences are dire when insulin and leptin production is compromised. Weight gain and other problems originate from the same core source as inflammation; unhealthy diets. Diets that include bread, cereals/ grains, pasta, rice, carbonated drinks, sugar-laden foods, and high concentrations of hydrogenated oils (trans fats) found in processed foods, fast foods, margarine, shortening, and some commercial peanut butter are ordained to create obesity and associated diseases.

Food options such as 'grains' may seem less obvious culprits, but rest assured they are equal offenders when it comes to contributing to poor nutrition and its effects. In fact, many prominent health experts consider grains to be "anti-nutrients" (plant compounds that reduce the body's ability to absorb essential nutrients), which contribute to leaky gut, cause inflammation, weaken the immune system, and trigger autoimmune disease (which is when your immune system, which defends your body against disease, decides your healthy cells are foreign and as a result, your immune system attacks healthy cells).

You may ask, "*So how did all these grains become such a large part of our diets?*" As mentioned earlier in the chapter, our ancient ancestors were hunter-gathers relying on animals, vegetables, and seasonal fruits for their nutrition. When humans discovered farming, the agriculture revolution was born, and we evolved from hunter-gatherers to farmers, with grains becoming the most prominent produce. The problem is, our hunter-gatherer bodies never adjusted properly to eating all these grains and that remains the case today.

Mark Sisson, author of the *Primal Blueprint* summarizes the condition perfectly:

> Grains have fundamentally altered the foods to which our species originally adapted over eons of evolutionary experience. For better or for worse, we are no longer hunter-gatherers. However, our genetic makeup is still that of a Paleolithic hunter-gatherer, a species whose nutritional requirements are optimally adapted to wild meats, fruits and vegetables, not to cereal grains. There is a significant body of evidence which suggests that cereal grains are less than optimal foods for humans and that the human genetic makeup and physiology may not be fully adapted to high levels of cereal grain consumption. We have wandered down a path toward absolute dependence upon cereal grains, a path for which there is no return.

Certain grain (and also some dairy) proteins mimic those found in viruses and bacteria, triggering an immune response when ingested. Gluten—the large, water-soluble protein that creates the elasticity in the dough (it's also the primary glue in wallpaper paste)—is found in most common grains, such as wheat, rye, and barley. Researchers now believe that as many as a third of us are probably gluten-intolerant or gluten-sensitive.

Grains also play a role in interference with vitamin D metabolism and related deficiencies of vitamins A, C, and B12. These nutrients are not present in grains (again, ironically, unless they have been processed and then "fortified" by adding back the missing vitamins—albeit at a much reduced bioavailability).

Ironically, the unprocessed—and, therefore, supposedly healthier "whole" grains are typically the highest in phytates (another antinutrient). Mineral deficiencies are common in underdeveloped nations that depend almost entirely on grain for their sustenance (bread accounts for 50 percent of the total calories consumed in at least half the countries in the world; some populations derive up to 80 percent of total calories from grain products).

There is sufficient evidence that this overreliance on grains—as well as on simple carb and sugar products in general—leads to numerous vitamin, mineral, and nutritional deficiencies. Most grains contain substances called phytates that easily bind to important minerals like calcium, magnesium, and zinc in the digestive tract, making them more difficult to absorb.

Anti-Nutrients – The Main Players

- Gluten
  All wheat, rye, and barley plants produce gluten. It is known to be one of the most difficult-to-digest plant proteins. Gluten is an

enzyme inhibitor that has become notorious for causing gastro-intestinal distress. Not only can gluten cause digestive problems, but it can contribute to leaky gut syndrome, autoimmune disease, allergic reactions, and cognitive problems as well.

The severe form of gluten sensitivity is Celiac's disease — but gluten is responsible for other less severe symptoms in a much larger percentage of people, including joint pain, headaches, fatigue, and poor memory.

Dr. David Perlmutter wrote in his book *Grain Brain*:

> Gluten, the protein found in wheat, barley, and rye is among the most inflammatory ingredients of the modern era. While a small percentage of the population is highly sensitive to gluten and suffers from celiac disease, it's possible for virtually everyone to have a negative, albeit undetected, reaction. Gluten sensitivity—with or without the presence of celiac—increases the production of inflammatory cytokines, which are pivotal players in neurodegenerative conditions and the brain is among the most susceptible organs to the deleterious effects of inflammation. I call gluten a "silent germ" because it can inflict lasting damage without your knowing it. While its effects might start with unexplained headaches and feeling anxious, or "wired and tired," they can worsen to direr disorders such as depression and dementia. Gluten is everywhere today, despite the gluten-free movement taking place even among food manufacturers.

In another of his renowned books - *Brain Maker*, Dr. Perlmutter observes:

> New research has come to light about the damaging effects of gluten on the microbiome. Indeed, it's quite possible that the entire cascade of adverse effects that takes place when the body is exposed to gluten starts with a change in the microbiome—ground

zero. Gluten's "sticky" attribute interferes with the breakdown and absorption of nutrients, which leads to poorly digested food that can then sound the alarm in the immune system, eventually resulting in an assault on the lining of the small intestine.

Phytates (Phytic Acid)

This is probably the most well-known anti-nutrient found in grains and legumes. It interferes with the absorption of minerals. Phytic acid can lock up high percentages of phosphorus, calcium, copper, iron, magnesium, and zinc. Some research indicates up to 80 percent of phosphorous found in high-phosphorus foods like pumpkin or sunflower seeds, along with 80 percent of zinc found in high-zinc foods like cashews and chickpeas, might be blocked by phytates. The same can be said for about 40 percent of magnesium-rich foods.

Phytic acid also interferes with calcium and iron absorption, raising the risk for health problems like anemia (iron deficiency) and bone loss. It inhibits certain essential digestive enzymes called amylase, trypsin, and pepsin. Amylase breaks down starch, while both pepsin and trypsin are needed to dissolve protein.

Lectins

In high quantities lectins found in beans and wheat, reduce nutrient absorption resulting in indigestion, bloating, and gas for many people. One of the most nutritionally significant features of plant lectins is their ability to survive digestion by the gastrointestinal tract. They can penetrate cells lining the digestive tract and cause a loss of gut epithelial cells, damage the membranes of the epithelium lining, interfere with nutrient digestion and absorption, stimulate shifts in the bacterial flora, and trigger autoimmune reactions. Lectins can cause gastrointestinal upset similar to food poisoning and immune responses like joint pain and skin rashes.

Saponins

Soy beans, chick peas, oats, quinoa, and plants similar to lectins produce saponins. Saponins affect the gastrointestinal lining contributing to leaky gut syndrome and autoimmune disorders. They're particularly resistant to digestion by humans and possess the ability to enter the bloodstream and trigger immune responses.

Omega-6; A Major Inflammation Culprit

Unfortunately, omega-6 fats are everywhere and almost unavoidable. We cook with them, bake with them, they are in most processed foods, fast food, and restaurant food. Subsequently, we are getting way too many of them!

Omega-6 fats are vegetable oils such as soybean oil, corn oil, safflower oil, sunflower oil, grape seed oil, peanut oil, and cotton seed oil. Margarine and shortening also are high in omega-6 amounts.

In the right amounts, omega-6 can be beneficial, but too much causes major inflammation throughout the body, including your arteries and immune system. Over- consumption of omega-6 decreases the body's ability to fight infections and diminishes the ability to find cancer-producing cells and rid the body of them before they cause cancer, increase inflammation, and atherosclerosis in the arteries.

The body constructs hormones from omega fatty acids. Hormones derived from the two classes of essential fatty acids have opposite effects. Those from omega-6 fatty acids increase inflammation (an important component of the immune response), blood clotting, and cell proliferation, while those from omega-3 fatty acids decrease those functions. Both families of hormones must balance to maintain optimum health, so there are some omega-6 benefits.

Many nutrition experts believe that before we relied so heavily on processed foods, humans consumed omega-3 and omega-6 fatty acids in roughly equal amounts. Now, to our great detriment, most North Americans and Europeans get far too much of the omega-6s and not enough of the omega-3s. This dietary imbalance may explain the rise of diseases like asthma, coronary heart disease, many forms of cancer, autoimmunity and neurodegenerative diseases, all of which are believed to stem from inflammation in the body. The imbalance between omega-3 and omega-6 fatty acids may also contribute to obesity, depression, dyslexia, hyperactivity, and even a tendency toward violence.

We will talk about countering Omega -6 with Omega-3 in the *Nutritional Intake* chapter.

Sugar, Artificial Sweeteners, and Diet Soda

As previously mentioned in this chapter, sugar, sugar-laden foods, and sweet sodas are major contributors to numerous health issues. A few of the more commonly known effects include; obesity, heart disease, Type 2 diabetes, gum disease, and tooth decay. Sugar interferes with immune function, causes major inflammation throughout the body, produces non-alcoholic liver disease, and is highly addictive as it causes a release of dopamine in the reward center of the brain.

Some of the lesser known effects might include contributing to plaque buildup in your arteries. Substances like sugar can oxidize and harden blood cholesterol. It accelerates aging when it hits the bloodstream by attaching itself to proteins; a process called glycation. These new molecular structures contribute to the loss of elasticity found in aging body tissues, from the skin to organs and arteries. The more sugar circulating in your blood, the faster resulting damage occurs.

Are we better off with artificial sweeteners and diet sodas? A recent study in mice showed that artificial sweeteners changed the gut bacteria of mice in ways that made them vulnerable to insulin resistance and glucose intolerance — both of which can lead to weight gain. Additional related research on mice suggests artificial sweeteners are associated with a drop in the appetite-regulating hormone leptin. Leptin is the hormone that inhibits hunger. (1)

Current study results on diet sodas published in the *Journal of the American Geriatrics Society* found that people who drank diet soda gained almost triple the abdominal fat over nine years as those who didn't drink diet soda. The study analyzed data from 749 people ages 65 and older surveyed every couple of years, questioned how many cans of soda they consumed a day, and how many of those sodas were diet or regular. (2)

The obvious conclusion is NO; we are NOT better off ingesting artificial sweeteners and diet sodas!

Overuse of Medications

A deadly pill culture has developed in the US. Studies indicate some 70% of the population is on some medication. The most commonly prescribed drugs are antibiotics, antidepressants, and pain suppressing opioids, according to research findings published in the journal *Mayo Clinic Proceedings*.

Americans account for 99 percent of the world's hydrocodone (Vicodin) consumption, 80 percent of the world's oxycodone (Percocet and OxyContin) consumption, and 65 percent of the world's hydromorphone (Dilaudid) consumption, according to the *New York Times*.

What's causing the epidemic overuse of drugs? It is something of a vicious cycle. Unhealthy lifestyle choices result in physical issues; doctors write copious prescriptions to deal with numerous conditions including, chronic pain, hypertension, heart failure, diabetes, infections, gastroesophageal reflux, and other overweight and obesity-related maladies.

While drugs serve the purpose of treating individual disorders they also contribute to poor health by promoting cellular toxicity, inflammation, accidental overdose, and even death.

Sedentary Behavior

The human body is designed for perpetual motion. For thousands of years, that's exactly what humans did -- MOVED. Survival was dependent on the ability to move. People moved to gather food, escape predators, and migrate to more desirable lands. As communities formed and conveniences advanced, humans remained in motion for long days of physical farm work and walking to destinations like school, social activities, or supplies. In the mid-20th century, technological advances began to rise. The universal availability of automation created a cultural shift from physically demanding work to office jobs eroding the requirements and benefits of physical activity.

Today, at a time when we have more choices than ever in almost every aspect of life, most people choose to be sedentary. Americans, for example, spend 93 percent of their lifetime indoors — and 70 percent of each day sitting. (3)

The World Health Organization associated the lack of physical activity with an estimated 3.2 million deaths a year and impacting the following:

- Heart Disease: Sitting for too long means your muscles aren't burning fat as they should causing blood to flow through the body at a slower pace and providing fatty acids the opportunity to clog the heart — leading to coronary heart disease. A study published in *Medicine & Science in Sports & Exercise* found the more time men spent in sedentary activities (sitting in cars, at desks, watching television), the more likely they were to develop cardiovascular disease.

- Diabetes: When you're not moving, your body isn't using as much blood sugar — and that's not a good thing. A study of more than 80,000 people found each hour they spent watching TV increased their risk of developing diabetes by 3.4 percent. "Netflix and chill" doesn't sound like such a desirable activity now, does it? Exercise is proven to be one of the most effective, natural treatments for diabetes, while a lack of physical activity is one of the leading causes for developing diabetes.
- Reduced Circulation: Remaining stationary for too long slows blood circulation to the legs, which can lead to swollen ankles, blood clots, swelling, and pain. A more dire complication from long bouts of sitting is deep vein thrombosis, the result of a blood clot forming in the legs. A blood clot can eventually break free and obstruct essential circulation in other parts of your body, including your lungs, heart, and brain.

- Fuzzy Thinking: Ironically, sitting down to work can lead to trouble concentrating. When we're not moving, there's less blood pumping throughout the body, including the brain. The lack of blood flow slows cognitive functions and leads to brain fog.

- Loss of Muscle and Bone Strength: Our bodies must maintain lean muscle tissue to perform daily tasks without damage. Living a sedentary lifestyle physically changes everything. Simple, routine events like shopping, running errands, even household chores become much more difficult. The reduction in motion is especially important in older adults, who are already losing muscle mass and bone strength.

Stress

The human body is designed to experience stress and react to it. Stress can be positive – as it can keep us alert and prepares us to avoid danger. Stress becomes a negative factor when a person faces continuous challenges without periods of relief or relaxation. As a result, individuals become overworked, and stress-related anxiety and illness can occur. Physical symptoms include headaches, upset stomach, elevated blood pressure, chest pain, and problems sleeping. Research suggests that stress can contribute to more serious, chronic symptoms and related diseases.

The use alcohol, tobacco, or drugs in an attempt to reduce stress symptoms serves to exacerbate the harmful results. Unfortunately, instead of relieving the stress and returning the body to a relaxed state, these toxic substances tend to keep the body in a stressed state causing greater physical problems.

A few examples of how stress can play havoc on our bodies include:

- Musculoskeletal System: The normal body reaction to stress is to tense muscles. Muscle tension is almost a reflex reaction to stress — it is the body's way of guarding against injury and pain. A sudden onset stress causes muscles to tense up all at once, and then release the tension when the stressful event passes. Chronic stress causes the muscles to remain in a constant state of guardedness. When muscles are taut and tense for long periods of time other reactions in the body are triggered promoting stress-related disorders. For example, both tension-type headaches and migraine headaches are associated with chronic muscle tension in the area of the shoulders, neck, and head.

- Respiratory System: Stress causes a person to breathe harder. That's not a problem for most people, but for individuals suffering from asthma or a lung disease such as emphysema, getting essential oxygen can be difficult. Some studies show that acute stress events — such as the death of a loved one — can trigger asthma attacks, in which the airway between the nose and the lungs constrict.

Rapid breathing associated with stress — or hyperventilation — can result in a panic attack in individuals prone to such occurrences.

- Cardiovascular: The heart and blood vessels comprise the two elements of the cardiovascular system that work together to provide nourishment and oxygen to the body's organs. The activity of the heart and blood also coordinates the body's response to stress.

- Acute Stress: Stress that is momentary or short-term such as meeting deadlines, being stuck in traffic, or suddenly slamming on the brakes to avoid an accident — causes an increase in the heart rate and stronger contractions of the heart muscle. The stress hormones — adrenaline, noradrenaline, and cortisol — act as messengers to signal these reactions. The vessels that direct blood to large muscles and the heart dilate, increase the amount of blood pumped to these parts of the body and elevates blood pressure. The effect is known as the "fight or flight" response. Once the acute stress episode has passed, the body returns to its normal state.

- Chronic Stress: Or a constant stress experienced over a prolonged period, can contribute to long-term problems for the heart and blood vessels. A consistent and ongoing increase in heart rate, and rising levels of stress hormones, and elevated blood pressure take a toll on the body. Long-term, ongoing stress can increase the risk for hypertension, heart attack, or stroke. Repeated acute stress and persistent chronic stress may also contribute to inflammation in the circulatory system, particularly in the coronary arteries, which is one pathway thought to link stress to a heart attack. It also appears that how a person responds to stress can affect cholesterol levels.

- Endocrine: When the body is stressed, the hypothalamus signals the autonomic nervous system and the pituitary gland starting the process to generate epinephrine and cortisol, sometimes called the "stress hormones." Stress signals from the hypothalamus cause the adrenal cortex to produce cortisol and the adrenal medulla to produce epinephrine initiating the process that provides the body with the energy to run from danger.

When cortisol and epinephrine are released, the liver produces more glucose, a blood sugar providing the fuel for "fight or flight" in an emergency. Most people don't use all of that extra energy, in which case the body can reabsorb the blood sugar, even if stress events occur again and again. But for some people — especially people vulnerable to Type 2 diabetes — that extra blood sugar can mean diabetes. Who's vulnerable? The obese and some ethnicities that are most inclined to diabetes, such as Native Americans.

- Gastrointestinal: People who are stressed tend to eat much more or much less than usual. If you eat more food or different types of food or increase the use of alcohol or tobacco, heartburn or acid reflux may occur. Stress or exhaustion can also increase the frequency and severity of heartburn pain.

  Stress causes the brain to send alert sensations in the stomach during stress. Your stomach can react with "butterflies," nausea, or pain. Severe stress can cause vomiting, diarrhea, or constipation. If stress becomes chronic, ulcers or severe stomach pain may develop. Stress affects what nutrients your intestines absorb and how quickly food moves through the body.

- Nervous System: The nervous system has several divisions; the central division involving the brain and spinal cord and the peripheral division consisting of the autonomic and somatic nervous systems. The autonomic nervous system (ANS) has a direct role in physical response to stress and is divided into the sympathetic nervous system (SNS), and the parasympathetic nervous system (PNS).

When the body is stressed, the SNS generates what is known as the "fight or flight" response. The body shifts all of its energy resources toward fighting off a threat or fleeing from an enemy. The SNS signals the adrenal glands to release hormones called adrenalin and cortisol. These hormones cause the heart to beat faster, respiration rate to increase, blood vessels in the arms and legs to dilate, the digestive process to change, and glucose levels (sugar energy) in the bloodstream to increase to deal with the emergency.

- Male Reproductive System: The male reproductive system is influenced by the nervous system. The parasympathetic part of the nervous system causes relaxation whereas the sympathetic part causes arousal. In the male anatomy, the autonomic nervous system also serves as a fight or flight response, producing testosterone and activating the sympathetic nervous system creating arousal.

Stress causes the body to release the hormone cortisol, which is produced by the adrenal glands. Cortisol is important to blood pressure regulation and the normal functioning of several body systems including cardiovascular, circulatory, and male reproduction. Excess amounts of cortisol can negatively affect the normal biochemical functioning of the male reproductive system.

Chronic stress or ongoing stress over an extended period can affect testosterone production, sperm production, maturation, and even cause erectile dysfunction or impotence. When stress affects the immune system, the body becomes vulnerable to infection. In the male anatomy, infections to the testes, prostate gland, and urethra affects normal male reproductive functioning.

- Female Reproductive System: Stress may affect menstruation among adolescent girls and women in several ways. For example, high levels of stress are associated with absent or irregular menstrual cycles, more painful periods, and changes in the length of cycles.

Stress may make premenstrual symptoms worse or more difficult to cope with and pre-menses symptoms may be stressful for many women. These symptoms include cramping, fluid retention, bloating, negative moods, (feeling irritable and "blue") and mood swings.

As menopause approaches, hormone levels fluctuate rapidly. The changes contribute to anxiety, mood swings, and feelings of distress. Thus, menopause can be a stressor in and of itself. Some of the physical discomforts associated with menopause, particularly hot flashes, can be difficult to control. Furthermore, emotional distress may worsen many of the physical symptoms.

Women juggle personal, family, professional, financial, and a broad range of other demands through-out their life. Stress, distraction, fatigue, and physical discomforts may reduce sexual desire — especially when women are simultaneously caring for young children or other ill family members, coping with chronic medical problems, feeling depressed, experiencing relationship difficulties or abuse, or dealing with work-related issues.

Studies show that if you learn how to manage stress, you can control blood sugar levels often with better success than with medication.

In Closing

I don't mean to paint a portrait of doom and gloom here, but I do think it is important to share the fact that our lifestyles are making us sicker, fatter, unhealthier, and they are aging us faster than nature intended. It's not too late for change my friends; you can make conscious choices to flip all of this around. In the coming chapters, I offer tools and solutions to combat everything mentioned. The entire program is intended to help achieve optimal wellness, reverse premature aging, and reveal a new vibrant, youthful you -- *The You Nature Intended*!

3

Nutritional Intake
(Secret 1)

"Let food be thy medicine and medicine be thy food."

~ HIPPOCRATES

Every principal discussed in this book is meant to work synergistically to support whole health. It cannot be overstated -- there is one single most important element involved with the process of reversing aging, improving overall health, and slowing the age-clock going forward. The critical piece of the holistic vitality is bound by what you put into your mouth.

I have tried numerous eating plans over the past thirty-plus years. Many of my ill-fated attempts were guided by the latest fads, current best-selling books, or publicity "hyped" nutritional discoveries of the time. Most of the adopted fashionable diet trends proved way off the mark as far as protecting what is truly healthy for our bodies. The biggest mistakes and misguided weight-loss trends of the past incorporated the 'fat-free' craze. The 'fat-free' movement failed to recognize just how important fat is to the human body. Followers ended up overcompensating for the lack of dietary fat by eating more carbs, ultimately creating, even more, propensity for obesity and associated health problems.

My recommendations are not influenced by the latest trends or fad diets. Through exhaustive reviews of respected research, personal experimentation and subsequent success, my suggested plans are based on what is biologically demonstrated to work most efficiently and effectively. I base my nutritional proposals on scientific data, personal trial and error – balanced with a little common sense.

Changes in diet can erase years from your physical appearance and improve overall health dramatically. A good diet increases energy, improves sleep, enhances skin tone and elasticity, clears foggy brains, supports weight loss, improves digestion, and decreases inflammation – as well as minimizing the achiness and puffiness that comes with it. My goal for you is to reveal the best 'you' nature intended; beautiful and healthy-inside-and-out. I want to help you improve the biological processes and restore your body to operating holistically as nature designed with an emphasis on vigorous, optimal brain function.

I would like to dispel a few myths and misnomers about food intake, and establish key practice points, before we explore the elements of your new living plan:

Carbohydrates

I have written about many of the problems associated with excessive carbohydrate consumption several times in the book. Changing a high-carb eating pattern is paramount in order to maximize the health and anti-aging benefits of my program. The critical key to the success of your new eating plan is moderating insulin production, which means you MUST eliminate or at the very least limit the intake of certain carbohydrates (sugars, bread, cereal, flour, rice, pasta, grains, etc.). I know it sounds challenging, but I promise once you get into the program you will see how easy the abstention becomes. The quality 'good' fats, proteins, and carbohydrates consumed completely satiates the appetite and hunger cravings for simple and processed carbs will dissipate.

As we go further into the chapter, I will detail the types of recommended carbohydrates.

Grains

I wrote quite extensively about the nutritional value (or lack thereof) of grains in the *Lifestyles* chapter and dispelled the idea that whole wheat or other whole grains are good for you. I examined the counterproductive aspects of grains; like their composition of plant toxins and anti-nutrients, and their contribution to digestion issues and inflammation. There are a few grain products that might be worth considering as a part of an anti-aging, healthy diet in moderation. Foods produced with sprouted grain or sourdough grain can be tolerated as both processes reduce the plant toxins and anti-nutrients, making them a little more digestible, and better able to release beneficial nutrients.

Fats

Fat has gotten a bad reputation over the years. Yes, some fats are not healthy (such as trans fats; margarine, shortening, and other hydrogenated oils as well as the over-consumption of pro-inflammatory omega-6 heavy vegetable oils; soybean oil, corn oil, safflower oil, sunflower oil, grape seed oil, peanut oil, and cottonseed oil). Those nutritional villains aside, we absolutely need fat in our diets, including some saturated fats -- in case you were wondering. Good fats are nutrient dense, rich in omega-3 fatty acids, and necessary for the absorption of minerals and conversion of other nutrients. They provide a concentrated source of energy, establish the building blocks for cell membranes and support a variety of hormones and hormone-like substances. Good fats boost satiety and they assist digestive function and slow absorption - promoting a sustained release of their nutrients.

In Paleolithic diets, our hunter-gatherer ancestors consumed omega-6 and omega-3 fats in a ratio of approximately 1:1. Today we consume almost twenty times* more omega-6 fats than our ancient ancestors and we've significantly reduced our intake of healthy, brain-boosting omega-3 fats. The ratio of omega-6 to omega-3 is important because the higher the ratio, the more omega-6, or the less omega-3, the more inflammation in the body.

One quick observation about omega-3; there is ample prominent scientific research correlating the increased consumption of brain-healthy omega-3 fatty acids to the threefold increase in the size of the human brain.

*This is in large part due to eating so many processed foods that contain omega-6 oils; our regular and high usage of these oils at home and in restaurants; most of our meat and dairy is derived from grain-fed animals instead of grass; and low consumption of wild, omega-3 rich fish.

Cholesterol

Right behind the bad fat myth is the claim cholesterol is equally dangerous. Nothing could be further from the truth. Cholesterol happens to be one of the most important substances in the human body. It is an important brain nutrient essential to facilitate synapses (connections) with other brain cells. Every cell membrane depends on cholesterol as a critical structural and functional component. Cholesterol acts as an antioxidant and a precursor to vital brain-supporting elements like vitamin D and essential hormones such as testosterone, estrogen, DHEA, cortisol, and pregnenolone. Most importantly, cholesterol is considered a principal fuel for the neurons.

Neurologist Dr. David Perlmutter writes in his acclaimed book *Brain Maker*:

> The brain demands high amounts of cholesterol as a source of fuel, but neurons cannot themselves generate significant amounts of it so they depend on cholesterol that is delivered by the bloodstream via a special carrier protein called LDL, or low-density lipoprotein. This is the same protein that is often demonized as being 'bad cholesterol.' [Scientifically,] there's nothing bad about LDL, which

is not a cholesterol molecule at all, good or bad. LDL is a vehicle for transporting life-sustaining cholesterol from the blood to the brain's neurons. It plays the fundamental role in the brain by capturing life-giving cholesterol and transporting it to the neuron, where it performs critically important functions.

Dr. Perlmutter goes on to say:

All of the latest science shows that when cholesterol levels are low, the brain simply doesn't function optimally. People with low cholesterol are at much greater risk for neurological problems from depression to dementia.

When cholesterol levels are low, the brain doesn't work well, and individuals are at a significantly increased risk for neurological problems as a consequence. But a caveat: Once free radicals damage the LDL molecule, it's rendered much less capable of delivering cholesterol to the brain. In addition to oxidation destroying the LDL's function, sugar can also render it dysfunctional by binding to it and accelerating oxidation. And when that happens, LDL is no longer able to enter the astrocyte, a cell charged with nourishing neurons. In the last ten years, new research has shown that oxidized LDL is a key factor in the development of atherosclerosis. The oxidized LDL particles get stuck in tiny crevices in the artery walls, creating plaques that then capture more cholesterol and other cellular particles. The plaques can then harden and restrict blood-flow, which is obviously not a good thing, but even worse is if one of the plaques breaks off and finds its way into the heart, which is certainly a possibility, that could be disastrous! We should therefore do everything we can to reduce the risk of LDL oxidation—not necessarily levels of LDL itself. A principal player in that risk of oxidation is higher levels of glucose; LDL is far more likely to become oxidized in the presence of sugar molecules that will bind to it and change its shape. Glycosylated proteins, which are the products of these reactions between proteins and sugar molecules, are associated with a fiftyfold increase in free radical formation as compared to non-glycosylated proteins. LDL is not the enemy. The problems occur when a higher-carbohydrate diet yields oxidized LDL and an increased risk of atherosclerosis. In addition, if and when LDL becomes a glycosylated molecule, it cannot present cholesterol to brain cells, and brain function suffers.

This latter part gives you a good idea of the real 'baddie' here. Sugar's role in causing cholesterol to oxidize and harden is irrefutable and if sugar weren't such a prominent part of the Western diet, we would not experience such major plaque buildup issues in the blood vessels or the brain.

PRELUDE

Our hunter/gatherer ancient ancestors ate from several nutrient dense wild food sources that included animal meats, fish, fruits, vegetables, and nuts and seeds. Notably absent from their diet were grains.

A 'normal' breakfast in the US today consists of bagels, muffins, toast, cereal, or donuts. We supplement that weak start with similarly processed food snacks throughout the day. None of these foods contribute any real nutritional value. Worse, they are loaded with bad carbs and calories, pro-inflammatory omega-6 fats, and they are composed of processed grains, all of which wreak havoc on your health.

Fundamentally, we must move away from the typical American or Western diet and onto a diet made up of nutrient dense foods; organic fruits and veggies, wild fish, free-range chicken, pasture eggs, and grass-fed meats and dairy. "Organic" foods, once only available at specialty retail outlets are becoming more and more available and affordable at local farmer's markets and food cooperatives. Healthier products may be a bit more expensive, but they are worth every penny. Think about the value you are ultimately adding to your body and the money saved by eliminating the need for medications to deal with the complications from a typical Western diet.

Most people discover a meal of healthier, organic foods is more appetizing and filling than commercially processed food. Thanks to their rich nutritional value, they make it almost impossible to overeat. To get the equal number of calories from a box of cereal or pack of Oreos, you would have to eat a few grocery bags full of broccoli and spinach. I admit a slight exaggeration, but you get the point. A meal consisting of the right protein, fat, and vegetables can keep you full and satiated for hours, while eating high-carb processed foods results in hunger and cravings soon after consumption. The consumption of high-carb, processed foods ultimately pitches the body into a perpetual pro-inflammatory, fat storing, and high/low energy state.

Our hunter-gatherer ancient ancestors ate when they were hungry and didn't eat when they were not. Sometimes they would go all day, or even days at a time, without finding food. There were no pastries, bags of chips, or boxes of cereal sitting around to munch. Fortunately, humans were designed to store fat for energy during times of hunger. Our bodies still burn fat for fuel. By consuming processed foods all day, we give our bodies more calories than they can process and our bodies end up storing the excess as fat. Overconsumption of food prevents the body from using any of its existing fat stores and causes it to keep storing more fat. It's a dangerous, complicated, vicious cycle when our body keeps getting the wrong food sources daily.

THE FOOD FUNDAMENTALS

Buy Organic, Grass-Fed, Pasture, and Wild Only

Macronutrients

Protein

Portion size should be about the size of your fist or a deck of cards for every meal. Sources for protein include grass-fed meats, pasture raised chicken, wild fowl, pasture eggs, fish and shellfish such as; salmon, halibut, black cod, mahi-mahi, grouper, herring, trout, sardines, anchovies, shrimp, crab, lobster, mussels, clams, oysters, as well as wild game, and wild fowl.

Fats

Quality fats include; avocados, organic cold pressed coconut oil, extra virgin olive oil, omega 3 from wild fish or high-quality triglyceride fish oil supplements, grass-fed butter, almonds, walnuts, Brazil nuts, macadamia nuts, and organic nut butters. (Coconut oil is especially good during the body's transition from carbs to fat as it is an efficient energy source and extra virgin olive oil is a great way to reduce inflammation as it is an omega-9, a cousin of omega-3. Do not overheat it though as that changes the chemical structure and it could lose its healthier properties).

Carbohydrates

- Vegetables: Eat as many dark green veggies as you like. Good sources of carbohydrates include; kale, spinach, chard, arugula, broccoli, asparagus, collard greens, Brussel sprouts, cauliflower, bok choy, green beans, and zucchini. Green, red, yellow, and orange bell peppers, cucumbers, onions, garlic, ginger, radishes and most herbs and spices can all be added into the program at liberty as well. You can have at least one portion of sweet potatoes, yams, turnips, butternut, acorn, pumpkin, or summer squash per day if you choose.

- Fruits: Try to keep fruit consumption to a maximum of 2-3 portions per day. Richly colored berries such as blueberries, blackberries, raspberries, and strawberries are preferred. Cantaloupe, honeydew melon, apples, pears, peaches, apricots, cherries, pineapple, grapes, oranges, tomatoes, and grapefruit are next down the list; and keep consumption of high sugar fruit such as bananas, papayas, and mangos to a minimum.

A general rule of thumb for fruits and vegetables: the richer, brighter, darker, and more vibrant the color, the more nutrient content it contains. This rule holds true for richly colored spices like turmeric and cinnamon as well. Many experts also estimate that organic fruits are ten times richer in major micronutrients than their conventional counterparts.

Brightly colored fruits and vegetables are rich in phytonutrients such as vitamins, minerals, flavonoids, antioxidants, phenols, and carotenoids offering a powerful first line of defense against oxidative damage from aging, stress, and inflammation. Moreover, antioxidants and other phytonutrients appear to contain cancer-fighting properties, support immune function, boost nutrient assimilation, and aid in digestion.

Cruciferous vegetables such as broccoli, Brussels sprouts, kale, arugula, turnips, bok choy, horseradish, cabbage, and cauliflower contain potent phytonutrients giving them anti-aging, anti-cancer, and antimicrobial properties. Packed with vitamins, minerals, antioxidants, fiber, cruciferous vegetables boost digestion functions. Garlic, onions, and ginger all have similar properties as well.

Micronutrients

Most organic fruits and vegetables have phytonutrients including concentrated amounts of vitamins, minerals, carotenoids, polyphenols, flavonoids, and antioxidants. As mentioned above, the deeper, brighter, richer colored fruits and vegetables tend to have higher nutrient values, especially antioxidants.

Although no longer used by the USDA, fruits, vegetables, herbs, tea, and spices were once measured for their antioxidant potency by Oxygen Radical Absorbance Capacity (ORAC) and the deep, rich, brightly colored foods always showed the highest antioxidant content. The USDA stopped 'officially' testing in 2012 and removed the ORAC database from its website claiming "ORAC values are routinely misused by food and dietary supplement manufacturing companies to promote their products."

The termination of the government's ORAC consumer information program is not surprising based on the misuse. To ensure you are getting what your body needs, antioxidants and most other nutrients should be derived from food intake. The assimilation level of nutrients in supplements is extremely low to non-existent while gaining nutrients from food sources is drastically higher. There are a few supplements that are proven nutritionally adequate, but for the most part, supplements are a waste of money. I will explain more in the *Supplements* chapter.

Interestingly, several studies have shown the ORAC values of cocoa powder, and dark chocolate are higher than those of virtually any fruit and they contain considerably more flavonoids than well-known sources like green tea and red wine. Even more good news -- all of these items are allowed in my program!

Sweeteners

I have highlighted the problems with most artificial sweeteners in other areas of the book. You may wonder about the use of other "natural" sweeteners like honey and agave nectar - both of which are promoted by many health-conscious consumers as superior alternatives? Unfortunately, honey has a similar effect on blood sugar levels as table sugar and agave contains a higher fructose concentration than even high fructose corn syrup (HFCS). Both products prompt undesirable insulin spikes and triglyceride production.

It is well-established that HFCS is more lipogenic (fat-promoting) than glucose because it is readily converted into either glucose or triglycerides in the liver. Diets high in HFCS substantially increase triglyceride levels, cause fatty-liver disease (the most common disease in America to-day, affecting 90 million Americans), and the risk of obesity, as well as Type 2 diabetes, heart attacks, strokes, cancer, and dementia.

Sugar

As a practice, eliminate sugar from your diet. The occasional sweet treat as indicated further in the chapter may be an exception. Do not add sugar to beverages or food and make reading product labels a habit. Avoid packaged products that contain sugar. Sugar is added to almost all processed foods be-cause it is a cheap way to improve taste and most people are addicted to sugar. You would be amazed at just how many extra grams of sugar you get every day from the typical America diet. For example: a bowl of Honey Nut Cheerios and one tablespoon of French vanilla coffee creamer contains a combined 28g of sugar. Eat a blueberry muffin and that adds another 35g of sugar. A 6-inch Subway sandwich and a bowl of tomato soup or a PBJ sandwich with a 6 oz. low-fat yogurt for lunch adds approximately 30g of sugar. Have a bowl of pas-ta with store-bought tomato sauce and a salad with 2 tablespoons of bottled dressing, or grilled chicken with 2 tablespoons of bottled barbecue sauce and a salad with candied walnuts - add 30g of sugar. Packaged granola bars contain 10-15 grams of sugar and a Snapple Peach Tea packs 39g of sugar. You can easily consume well over a 100g of sugar per day nibbling on common, pack-aged foods without even knowing it. Sugar-laden foods greatly stress insulin sensitivity and reinforce the addiction to both sugar and all simple carbs. It is not difficult to understand why obesity and Type 2 diabetes are at epidemic levels among all age groups in the US and other Western countries.

Dairy

I recommend dairy consumption, but it must be produced by 100% or-ganic, grass-fed animals. Considering those who are lactose intolerant, you should leave dairy out of your diet. For all others, as long as you stay with 100% organic, grass-fed, whole-milk dairy products such as milk, yogurt, kefir, cheese, you will attain a lot of nutrients from the products.

Yoghurt and kefir improve gut health, and both products are high in probiotics. It is important to stress that buying low-fat or no-fat versions of such products is a waste of money. The primary beneficial nutrients are in the fat, so ONLY buy the whole-milk versions. Also, only buy unsweetened/unflavored varieties of these products as the others contain sugar/sweeteners/colorants/flavorings. Unsweetened yogurts and kefir products are delicious on their own but if you find the taste difficult to adjust to, try adding fresh organic berries or other types of fruits.

Avoid any variety of grain fed dairy as it is high in omega 6 fatty acids and we already consume too much of them in our diets. Grain fed animal products primarily come from concentrated animal feeding operations (CAFO). I will explain a little further on why CAFOs should be avoided. Remember, if the label doesn't say "100%, grass-fed," it isn't. If you can't get 100% grass-fed dairy don't bother including dairy in your diet, with the exception of small amounts of organic unsweetened kefir or yogurt for their probiotics.

Omega 3

Omega 3 fatty acids are essential fatty acids (a fatty acid that is essential to human health, but cannot be manufactured in the body and must be obtained through dietary intake). In modern diets, there are few sources of omega-3 fatty acids. The fat of cold water fish such as; salmon (Sockeye contains the highest followed by Coho and King), sardines, herring, mackerel, black cod, and bluefish or from plant foods such as walnuts, flax seeds, chia seeds, hemp seeds, and leafy green vegetables like spinach, kale, and algae are all good sources for the nutrient.

There are three forms of Omega 3 fatty acids. Two of the three forms of Omega 3's are critical for the human body to function properly; docosahexaenoic acid (DHA), and eicosapentaenoic acid (EPA). The third Omega 3 is alpha-linolenic acid (ALA). Studies have shown that DHA and EPA are the most beneficial forms of Omega 3 fatty acids. These essential elements are easily assimilated by the body and deliver efficacies faster. ALA is converted into DHA and EPA in the body, but the process is very inefficient and the absorption is at a very low ratio. This means that even if you consume large amounts of ALA, your body can only convert a relatively small amount into DHA and EPA, and only when there are sufficient enzymes to do so. While ALA will produce results, it takes a great deal longer than DHA/EPA. (1)

The best sources of DHA and EPA are fatty, cold water fish and algal oil. High quality, triglyceride form fish oils (more on this in the *Supplement* chapter), shellfish, and fish eggs also produce DHA and EPA.

DHA and EPA have numerous health benefits, including tremendous anti-inflammatory properties. They have shown to be as effective as non-steroidal anti-inflammatory drugs (NSAID) such as aspirin, Ibuprofen, Naproxen, and Celecoxib at reducing inflammation. DHA and EPA block inflammatory cytokines and prostaglandins and they are converted by the body into powerful anti-inflammatory chemicals called resolvins and pro-tectins. (2, 3, 4).

I stress, inflammation is a major contributor to poor health and prema-ture aging and one of the key areas targeted in my anti-aging program. You will not begin looking or feeling your best if there is internal inflammation causing puffy, saggy skin and aches and pains all over the body.

The ability to act as anti-inflammatories positions DHA and EPA as very effective factors in the treatment and prevention of hundreds of medi-cal conditions. They support heart health as well as normal growth and development of the brain. The human brain is made of 20% DHA, which must be replenished regularly. DHA and EPA both generate neuroprotec-tive metabolites. In double-blind, randomized, controlled trials, DHA and EPA combinations have been shown to benefit attention deficit/hyperac-tivity disorder (ADHD), autism, mood disorders, dyspraxia, dyslexia, and they have been linked to lower dementia and improved focus and memory.

They have also been effective in treatment of various types of cancer, arthritis, and infertility. (5, 6, 7, 8)

Need any more reasons to eat more of the right Omega-3s?

Probiotic foods

Probiotic foods provide another HUGE piece to optimal aging efforts. Keeping the gut healthy rewards with long-term benefits. Failure to take care of proper digestion brings on many detrimental side-effects.

Diet and lifestyle choices play a critical role in gut health. Research has uncovered an intricate web connecting our gut flora to virtually every process in the body. Imbalances in our microbial communities are implicated in countless health issues including immune disorders, psychological distress, and many other chronic health problems of our times. There is more information about gut functioning in the *Healthy Gut – Healthy Brain* chapter.

I recommend the consumption of probiotic-rich foods every day. These super foods include:

- Yogurt: An explosion of yogurt brands has taken over the grocery dairy section. Educate yourself about which brands to buy; many of them—both Greek and regular—are loaded with added sugar, artificial sweeteners, and artificial flavors. Read the labels. People with dairy sensitivities may find coconut yogurt is an excellent dairy-free way to work plenty of enzymes and probiotics into the diet. I personally only eat organic grass-fed, unsweetened/unflavored whole milk yogurt, which I have already recommended to you earlier in this chapter. The brands I buy include Maple Hills Creamery, Traderspoint Creamery, Organic Valley, and Stonyfield. There may be other local brands available in your area, but these are the prominent, reputable brands where I live.

- Kefir: Similar to yogurt, this fermented dairy product is a unique combination of milk and fermented kefir grains. Kefir has been consumed by humans for well over 3,000 years. The term "kefir" originated in Russia and Turkey and translated it means "feeling good." Kefir has a slightly acidic, tart flavor and contains an estimated 10 to 34 strains of probiotics and overall, significantly more than yogurt. People sensitive to dairy may also find coconut kefir an option. I trust the same brands of kefir as the yogurt products mentioned. I don't buy very much kefir because I make my own. My DIY kefir delivers a much higher probiotic content (trillions of CFUs more) as well as more strains than the shelf assortment available in stores. Kefir in general contains a wider array of microorganisms than yogurt and kefir produces an enzyme that digests lactose. To make kefir buy kefir grains (from Amazon or health stores) and follow the instructions. My method is simple:

  1. Add kefir grains to grass-fed, whole milk in a large mouth glass jar
  2. Place a double layer paper-towel over the jar's mouth
  3. Secure the paper towel with a rubber band
  4. Store jar in a cool cupboard for 24 hours
  5. Strain formula through a sieve before consuming
  6. Re-submerge kefir grains in liquid to keep them active.

- Kimchi: Delivers essential bacteria plus, kimchi is also an excellent source of calcium, iron, beta-carotene, and vitamins A, C, B1, and B2. I recommend organic, fresh, raw variants in the refrigerated sections of stores like Whole Foods.

- Sauerkraut: This fermented cabbage is full of fuel healthy gut bacteria. It also contains choline, a chemical needed for the proper transmission of nerve impulses from the brain through the central nervous system. Organic, raw sauerkraut, is usually in the refrigerator sections of food stores.

- Pickles: One of the easiest and most popular natural probiotics are pickles. For many, pickles can become the gateway food to other, more exotic fermented foods. Interestingly, pickles is a food pregnant women often crave. Choose a smaller food manufacturer that uses organic products and read labels to avoid purchasing pickles that are full of sugar. Try to stick to the salted versions.

- Pickled Fruits and Vegetables: Pickling fruits and veggies, such as carrot sticks, green beans, asparagus, and okra transforms the usual into the extraordinary. Whether you do this yourself or buy pickled produce, keep in mind, the probiotic benefits are only present in unpasteurized foods pickled in brine, not vinegar.

- Kombucha Tea: Originating in Japan, it is a form of fermented black tea consumed for centuries. Kombucha tea is effervescent, and its primary health benefits include digestive support, increased energy, and liver detoxification.

- Tempeh: This fermented soybean product came from Indonesia. It is another good source of probiotics. Tempeh is created by adding a tempeh starter to soybeans. The product is then left to sit for a day or two. The result is a cake-like product that may be eaten raw or by boiling it with miso. Tempeh may be used as a substitute for meat in a stir-fry meal. Do not eat deep-fried tempeh, which is often how it is prepared and served in restaurants.

- Miso: Miso is a traditional Japanese spice found in many traditional foods. It is created by fermenting soybean, barley or brown rice with koji. Koji is a fungus, and the fermentation process takes anywhere from a few days to a few years to process. Miso can be made into a delicious soup or spread on crackers in place of butter, or on vegetables as a spread.

- Brine-Cured Olives: Olives that are brine-cured are an excellent source of probiotics. For the maximum health effects, be sure to select a product that is organic first. Next, be certain that your olives aren't produced by a huge, commercial manufacturer. Choose a smaller company that advertises probiotics. Also, make sure that the olives do not contain sodium benzoate.

- Fermented Meat, Fish, and Eggs: Pickled meats, fish, and eggs are available in many natural, organic, and gourmet food shops. They are delicious and highly recommended.

Consumers spend thousands of dollars on a variety of nutritional supplements including probiotics. I am not a fan of probiotic supplements. Many supplements do not contain ingredients as advertised. The reality is, even if they were made with the displayed label list, most of the essential elements could not survive harsh stomach acids in to get to the intestines. Therefore, it is impossible to get the efficacy by depending on supplements, which renders them a waste of money in my book. My advice is to introduce probiotics to your body by what you eat and drink. By ingesting healthy, probiotic-rich foods you are guaranteed colony-forming units (CFU) of bacteria as well as the efficacies from them, plus food sources are much cheaper than supplements.

Dr. Joseph Mercola from *Mercola.com* states:

> Fermented foods not only give you a wider variety of beneficial bacteria, they also give you far more of them, so it's a much more cost-effective alternative to supplements. Here's a case in point; It is unusual to find a probiotic supplement containing more than 10 billion colony-forming units. But when my team actually tested fermented vegetables produced by probiotic starter cultures, they had 10 trillion colony-forming units of bacteria. Literally, one

serving of vegetables was equal to an entire bottle of a high potency probiotic! So clearly, you're far better off using fermented foods.

Seems like a no-brainer right?

Why Grass-Fed Products?

The natural diet for animals such as cattle, bison, goats, and sheep is grass and shrubs -- not grains. When left to their own devices, cattle will not graze on corn or soybeans. Transitioning these animals to grain is motivated by money as it is easier to fatten livestock up on the bulkier feed, so the time from farm to market is dramatically reduced. The problem with this equation is the minimal consideration for producing the best nutritional value for consumers.

Grains are as hard for animals to digest and process as they are for humans. A diet of grain can make the animal sick, necessitating a constant flow of interventive antibiotic treatments. Poor gut health in animals promotes disease. Antibiotics and hard to digest feed radically alter the bacterial balance and composition in the animal's gut.

Concentrated animal feeding operations (CAFO) fatten cows for slaughter in gigantic feedlots. They bulk as quickly as possible with the help of grains and growth-promoting drugs and antibiotics. When you eat CAFO beef, you are consuming small amounts of antibiotics and other drugs in each bite. Regularly consuming even small doses of antibiotics is a surefire way to destroy your gut health, which in turn will have a detrimental effect on your overall health and immune function. The condition makes you more susceptible to chronic disease and increases susceptibility to antibiotic-resistant infections.

The antibiotics used by CAFOs is detectible in an alarming amount of the meat sold in U.S. supermarkets and restaurants. The meat contains high levels of antibiotic-resistant bacteria (superbugs), which can spread antibiotic-resistance. The saturation of antibiotics threatens to create a post-antibiotic era where necessary medicines, critical to treating seriously ill people may become ineffective. Superbugs cause infections that are harder to treat and more likely to result in health complications or death. (9)

Organic, grass-fed standards, on the other hand, do not permit non-medical use of antibiotics. With antibiotic-resistant disease being a major public health hazard, buying organic and grass-fed meats and dairy is an important consideration in more ways than one.

Altering the animals' diet from grass to grain affects the nutritional composition of the meat and dairy products derived from them. Let's have a closer look at why grass-fed meat and dairy are far superior to grain:

"Grass-fed" products may not be a familiar term to all consumers. Products that are labeled "100% grass-fed" come from animals that have grazed in pastures year-round, rather than being fed a processed grain diet for much of their lives. Grass feeding improves the quality of nutrients in meats and dairy products making them richer in: omega-3 fats, vitamin B12, B3, B6, E, and A, beta-carotene, magnesium, calcium, potassium, iron, zinc, phosphorus, sodium, creatine, and carnosine. They are especially loaded with Conjugated Linoleic Acid (CLA), a type of fat associated with a wide variety of health benefits, including immune and inflammatory system support, improved bone mass, improved blood sugar regulation, reduced body fat, reduced risk of heart attack, and maintenance of lean body mass. (10)

The amount of CLA in meat and dairy products tends to increase exponentially with the consumption of fresh grasses by cattle. Cows exposed to ample supplies of fresh pasture produced increased amounts of CLA. The CLA content of meat and dairy from 100% grass-fed cattle is typically 300-500% higher than meat and dairy from conventionally fed cows. (11)

Studies indicate grass-fed cows have significantly more omega-3's and conjugated linoleic acid (CLA) than grain fed beef. One study highlighted that 80 days of grain feeding was enough to destroy the omega-3 content of the researched beef. CLA content plummeted in the same timeframe. The longer the animals were fed grains, the lower the quality of their meat. (12)

Health Benefits of Grass-fed Butter

In countries where cows are grass-fed, butter consumption is associated with a dramatic reduction in heart disease risk. As we have established, grass-fed products are significantly more nutrient-dense than their grain-fed counterparts, and these nutrients are incredibly important for the heart. (13, 14)

According to an Australian led study; cows were grass-fed, the research individuals who ate the most high-fat dairy from the test animals had a 69% lower risk of death from cardiovascular disease, compared to those who ate the least. (15)

Several other studies from countries where cows are largely grass-fed (like many European countries) agree with the Australian data - high-fat dairy products are associated with a reduced risk of heart disease. (16, 17, 18)

Grass-fed butter is also loaded with vitamin K2, the scarce nutrient that de-calcifies arteries. In case you haven't heard of it, vitamin K is one of the most important nutrients for optimal heart health. There are several forms of the vitamin: K1 (phylloquinone) is found in plant foods like leafy greens; K2 (menaquinone) is found in animal foods. Although the two forms are structurally similar, they appear to have different effects on the body. K1 is important in blood clotting; vitamin K2 helps to keep calcium out of your arteries. High-fat dairy products from grass-fed cows are among the best dietary sources of vitamin K2. (19, 20, 21)

Finally, I wrote about inflammation in the *Lifestyles* chapter being at the root of disease. One of the many areas affected by inflammation is the heart and inflammation is believed to be a leading driver of heart disease. It is proven, inflammation in the endothelium (lining of arteries) is a crucial part of the pathway that ultimately leads to plaque formation and heart attacks. One nutrient that appears to be able to fight this inflammation is called butyrate* (or butyric acid). Butyrate is a short-chain saturated fatty acid that studies show is an excellent anti-inflammatory, which helps reduce the risk of heart disease. (22, 23, 24, 25, 26, 27)

*This health-promoting fatty acid is only found in a few foods and butter is one of them. I have cited many positive health reasons to choose grass-fed products. One of the best consideration is grass-fed butter, which contains significantly higher levels of butyrate than grain-fed (standard) butter.

Farmed Fish Anyone?

Like the CAFOs for the production of meat and dairy products, farmed fish falls pretty much in the same category. It's a frustrating paradox for consumers who choose fish for their health sake. The nutritional benefits of fish are greatly decreased when it is farmed. Consider omega-3 fatty acids; wild fish get their omega-3's from eating aquatic plants. Farmed fish, however, are often fed corn, soy, or other feedstuffs that contain little or no omega-3's. This unnatural, high-grain diet means some farmed fish accumulate unhealthy levels of the wrong fatty acids.

Farmed fish are packed in confined areas, creating very unnatural and unhealthy conditions. They are raised in feces-filled, septic tanks. Fish farms are rife with toxins, diseases, and parasites, prompting operators to fight back by dumping concentrated antibiotics and other chemicals into the water. The practice has serious, far-reaching effects on consumers causing antibiotic-resistant disease strains, and a devastating impact on local ecosystems.

Eat ONLY wild caught fish.

Alkalinity/Acid Balance

The successful balance of alkalinity and acidity is paramount to optimizing my program.

Consuming processed foods, sugars, grains (wheat, corn, rice, pasta, breads, cereals, etc.), deep-fried foods, heavy amounts of alcohol and caffeine, cigarettes, carbonated drinks, and artificial sweeteners cause excess acidity in the body. Over-the-counter medications and prescription drugs also promote an acidic imbalance in the body, a precursor of many health problems and disease.

Emphasizing alkaline-forming food such as vegetables, fruits, nuts, and seeds in your diet can optimize the acid/base balance. Alkaline-forming foods serve to improve overall internal health while reducing your susceptibility to environmental and dietary toxins.

Plant foods naturally promote a beneficial balance between acidity and alkalinity in the bloodstream. Almost all cells prefer a slightly alkaline environment to function properly, but many metabolic processes, including the normal production of cellular energy, resulting in the release of acidic waste products. The buildup of acidic waste is toxic to the body and causes all sorts of health issues, including regular heartburn and acid reflux. So, your body works very hard at all times to preserve a slightly alkaline environment, measured by "pH" levels. Our bodies have evolved several highly refined buffering systems to balance the pH. Ingesting acid-producing foods makes it that much more difficult to achieve optimal pH homeostasis.

Examples of foods that promote alkalinity include; root vegetables such radishes, beets, carrots, turnips, horseradish, and rutabaga; cruciferous vegetables, broccoli, cabbage, cauliflower, Brussel sprouts, collard greens, arugula, and bok choy; leafy greens kale, chard, turnip greens, spinach, and almonds. Garlic introduces numerous other health benefits in addition to alkalinity.

Cayenne peppers (capsicum) are a part of a family of potent, tropical peppers which contain enzymes essential to endocrine function; cayenne is among the most alkalizing foods. It is known for its antibacterial properties and is a rich supply of vitamin A, making it a helpful agent in fighting off the harmful free radicals that lead to stress and illness. Lemons - may be the most alkalizing food of all. I like to add a squeezed half of a lemon to my tea in the morning and at night.

Bone Broth

You may ask, *"What is bone broth?"* This little anti-aging secret has recently become a new health and wellness buzzword. Bone broth delivers many incredible nutritional and health benefits well worth considering. Bone broth is an ancient food ingrained in traditional cultures for its super health and wellness value. The extensive contribution of bone broth spreads throughout the body, making it a health food staple that you should absolutely keep in your kitchen.

1. Body Support: Bone broth, by the very nature of its creation, contains collagen. Collagen is a protein matrix inside the bones, tendons, ligaments and other flexible tissues. It is broken down during the cooking process to form a gelatin substance, which is very easy for our bodies to digest and assimilate. Collagen plays a vital role in support of skin, nails, and hair health. Bone broth also contains other vital nutrients including chondroitin sulfates, glucosamine, and similar joint health substances that boost good health.

2. Nutrient Absorption: According to *Wellness Mama.com, a website dedicated to wholesome food choices and nutritional advice,* bone broth plays a vital role in nutrient absorption. It is a reliable source of

bio-available nutrients and offers an amino-acid structure and high-gelatin content making it healing and soothing for your gut. According to Jill Grunewald, author, holistic nutritional coach, and founder of *Healthful Elements*, a holistic nutrition practice, cited in an article by *Shape.com*, the gelatin found in the bone broth can help to seal holes in the intestines to hold food intolerances, cure chronic diarrhea, constipation, and other digestive issues.

3. Amino Acids: Bone broth, is an excellent source for a number of essential amino acids. This is important due to the fact amino acids are typically difficult to integrate into an ordinary diet. Introducing amino acids into the body through other sources is vital. These absorbent amino acids include arginine, glycine, proline, and glutamine.

4. Immune Health and Gut Health: *Wellness Mama* makes a good point about wholesome chicken soup. Chicken soup has long been respected for its important role in remedying illness, but the benefits have not been fully understood until recently. Research studies are beginning to unravel the fact that broth plays a vital role in the immune system, especially when it comes to the gut. Broth packs a high collagen and gelatin content which lends support to the gut. It also possesses a high amino acid content which aids in the reduction of inflammation during the healing process.

According to Dr. Campbell McBride author of *Gut and Psychology Syndrome*, gelatin can help to "*Heal and Seal*" the gut, making it particularly helpful in reversing what is known as the leaky gut syndrome as well as other digestive problems. (28, 29, 30, 31, 32, 33)

Different Types of Broths - Bone broth is not the same as regular broth, and neither is it the same as traditional stock. Understanding the differences is important, because each can offer different nutritive benefits, especially in different quantities. Each have vastly different flavors, especially when produced from different animals. Here is a brief rundown on the three most common broths:

- Bone Broth: Bone broth is made with animal bones and contains a small amount of meat, whatever adheres to the bones. The bones are roasted and then simmered for at least 24 hours, removing minerals and nutrients from the bones and releasing them into the broth. Ultimately, so many of the nutrients leave the bones during the cooking process that the bones fall apart with applied pressure.

- Broth: Regular broth is made from the meat but may contain a small amount of bone, and the broth is typically only simmered for a short time period. The flavor is much lighter than with bone broth, because the broth is cook from just the meat without the bones, but also because the meat is simmers for a much shorter time.

- Stock: Stock like bone broth, is made using the bone and may also contain a small quantity of meat. The bones are typically roasted prior to simmering to improve the flavor. The stock is simmered for several hours rather than days to produce mineral- and gelatin-rich fluids.

Broths, stocks and bone broths all produce fluids that are rich in nutrients, but bone broths produce the most nutrient-dense liquids because they cook the nutrient-rich bones for the longest time. It is for this reason that bone broth is gaining popularity for its nutritional benefits.

I only buy grass-fed bones from cattle or bison, pasture raised chicken bones or use the remaining carcass after roasting and eating an organic pasture raised chicken or turkey. I also recommend making bone broth from organic pasture raised chicken feet, which contains even higher levels of collagen.

A Little More on Cholesterol and Carbs

This section will detail how your daily diet should be structured. You will undoubtedly notice the scarcity of simple carbohydrates, which we have established ARE NOT GOOD FOR YOU! Once you digest the information, you will understand how carbs can affect cholesterol and what makes this so dangerous.

A healthy eating plan marrying the combination of low carbs and good fats, along with exercise, will generally raise HDL, lower both triglycerides, small and dense LDL, and prevent heart disease, regardless of your genetic predisposition.

HDL is effective at scavenging oxidized cholesterol from LDL in the bloodstream… if your HDL is high, it's much less likely you'll encounter a heart disease problem. Cholesterol is fat-soluble, but it must travel to and from cells in the watery environment of the bloodstream. It must be transported by special spherical particles called lipoproteins. There are several varieties of lipoproteins with different transporting functions such as chylomicrons, LDL, IDLs, HDLs, and VLDLs (low-density, Intermediate-density, high-density, and very low-density lipoproteins). Each of these lipoproteins carries a certain percentage of cholesterol, triglycerides, and other minor fats. Blood test values for triglycerides and HDL, LDL, and VLDL cholesterol represent the combined total in the bloodstream of what all the lipoproteins are transporting.

VLDLs, the largest of the cholesterol complexes, are manufactured in the liver in the presence of high levels of triglycerides (triglycerides are also made in the liver—from excess carbohydrates and fats). Hence, VLDLs comprise 80 percent triglyceride (and a little cholesterol). After leaving their birthplace in the liver, these lipoproteins deliver their cargo to fat and muscle cells for energy. Once these VLDLs have deposited their triglyceride load inside a fat or muscle cell, the size decreases substantially, and they become LDLs. At this point, they exhibit mostly cholesterol and a little bit of remaining triglyceride. In a healthy person, most of these LDL molecules are called "large fluffy" or "buoyant" LDLs. As such, they are generally harmless, even at relatively high levels, as they go about their assigned task of delivering cholesterol to the cells that need it.

The real trouble starts when triglycerides are unusually high in the bloodstream. This condition occurs routinely by consuming a high-carb diet which boosts insulin production.

Excessive insulin is also now considered a central catalyst in the development of atherosclerosis. Insulin promotes platelet adhesiveness (sticky platelets clot more readily) and the conversion of macrophages (a type of white blood cell) into foam cells, which are the cells that fill with cholesterol and accumulate in arterial walls. Eventually, a cholesterol and fat-filled "tumor" blocks circulation in the artery, a situation further aggravated by increased platelet adhesiveness and thickness of the blood. In addition, insulin reduces blood levels of nitric oxide (a compound that relaxes the endothelium, the lining of your arteries), causing the artery walls to become more rigid. This drives up blood pressure and increases the sheer force of blood against the arterial wall, further exacerbating the atherosclerotic condition. The entire process induces massive inflammation, which we have established at many points in the book is NOT GOOD FOR YOU.

More about the benefits of carbs reduction in the *Weight Loss* chapter.

MENU IDEAS

The following menu ideas provide examples of the variety of meals you can make at home. Ideally, they induce some creativity and inspire numerous menus for your family. The sky is the limit here! Abundant food types are included in this plan so it is up to you to find fun and interesting ways to eat them.

Breakfast

- Omelet* made with three pasture eggs (omega 3 and/or organic acceptable), add vegetables, mushrooms, peppers, onions, and tomatoes; cheese; avocado; turkey meat; salsa and ¼ cup of blueberries

- Two-three scrambled eggs* with 1-ounce cheddar cheese and sautéed veggies (onions, mushrooms, spinach, broccoli)

- Three-four slices of lox or smoked salmon with 1-ounce goat cheese, sliced tomatoes and a half of an avocado.

- Sausage and 2-3 eggs (grass-fed sausage) *

- Two poached eggs and a half of an avocado drizzled with extra virgin olive oil with an optional fresh squeeze of lemon juice and a touch of salt and pepper or 2 tablespoons of salsa.

- 1-cup yogurt topped with fresh berries, a small handful of almonds or walnuts, and shaved organic, unsweetened coconut.

- Two-three soft-sautéed eggs with grated cheese and salsa (use either homemade salsa or if it is store bought one check for added sugars in it).

- 1-cup grass-fed whole milk-based kefir, an apple, and a small handful of raw organic almonds, walnuts, or Brazil nuts.

*See cooking method options as well as 'fast' options at the end of this section.

Lunch

- Mixed salad greens - Try to stick to dark, richly colored greens such as spinach, kale, arugula, chard, collard greens. Add a variety of additional vegetables such as carrots, jicama, red peppers, cherry tomatoes (small handful) and grilled or shredded chicken (approximately 3 ounces), and an optional tablespoon of chopped nuts or seeds. Add a few tablespoons of homemade, extra virgin olive oil and balsamic vinegar (choose a good quality-low sugar version) or lemon juice dressing, seasoned with salt and pepper and herbs if desired. The chicken may be substituted with beef, shrimp, or grilled fish, canned tuna, salmon, or sardines. This is a general salad idea. Use some creativity and make different types. Important to stay with a clean dressing and avoid store bought.

- Grilled* or sautéed* chicken breast basted with mustard, olive oil, and lemon, or balsamic vinegar, herbs and spices. Add a side of leafy greens dressed with sautéed balsamic vinegar and olive oil.

- Grilled or sautéed sockeye salmon with lemon butter and a side of leafy greens dressed in balsamic vinegar and olive oil.

- Grass-fed beef/bison or chicken/turkey burger wrapped in lettuce (no bun) dressed with tomato, onion, served with a small deep orange (Jewel) sweet potato with grass-fed butter or virgin cold pressed coconut oil.

- Grilled grass-fed steak with a side of roasted, steamed, or stir-fried vegetables.

- Can of sardines, half an avocado, and sauerkraut or kimchee.

- Charcuterie – cold meats (good quality such as those from Whole Foods deli – no processed cold-cuts), grass-fed cheeses, raw veggies and hummus dip.

- Bone broth with added protein of choice, chopped onions, bell peppers, tomatoes, and celery.

*See cooking method options as well as 'fast' options at the end of this section.

Dinner

- Grilled*, sautéed*, or broiled grass-fed (cut of your choice) steak, and mixed vegetables sautéed in butter and garlic.

- Sautéed wild salmon with steamed asparagus, zucchini and small deep orange (Jewel) sweet potato with grass-fed butter or virgin cold pressed coconut oil.

- Grilled, sautéed, or roasted chicken, with steamed green vegetables.

- White wine and butter baked* wild fish with steamed vegetables zucchini and small deep orange (Jewel) sweet potato with grass-fed butter or virgin cold pressed coconut oil.

- Roasted* lemon and olive oil basted grass-fed Lamb with unlimited green beans and broccoli.

- Homemade meatloaf using grass-fed ground beef, onions, bell peppers, eggs, and few tablespoons of coconut flour instead of bread crumbs. Steamed broccoli, asparagus, or spinach on the side.

- Grass-fed beef stew made with bone broth, carrots, onions, celery, bell peppers, red wine, and herbs and spices. Mixed green salad on the side.

- Stir-fried vegetables with sliced protein of your choice and herbs and spices to taste.

*See cooking method options as well as 'fast' options at the end of this section.

Beverages

- Water: Drink purified, chlorine-free water (preferably reverse osmosis water). Chlorinated water has a negative effect on gut bacteria and actually kills good bacteria in the gut.

- Tea: Organic, unsweetened green*, black*, and herbal teas. Do not add sugar, sweeteners, or creamer. If you choose to add a creamer to your tea, use grass-fed whole milk or cream only.

*The polyphenols in tea, which include EGCG (epigallocatechin gallate) and many others, have been found to offer protection against many types of cancer. The polyphenols in green tea may constitute up to 30 percent of the dry leaf weight, so, when you drink a cup of green tea, you're drinking a fairly potent solution of healthy tea polyphenols. Green tea is the least processed kind of tea, so it also contains the highest amounts of EGCG of all tea varieties. Keep in mind, however, that many green teas have been oxidized, and this process may take away many of its valuable properties. The easiest sign to look for when evaluating a green tea's quality is its color: if your green tea is brown rather than green, it's likely been oxidized.

I primarily buy matcha green tea because it contains the entire ground tea leaf, and can contain over 100 times the EGCG provided from regular brewed green tea. I recommend you do so as well.

- Coffee (optional): Do not use as coffee an energy crutch and don't add sugar, sweetener, or creamer. If you choose to add creamer, use grass-fed whole milk, half & half or cream only.

- Wine (optional): Consumption of one or two glasses (preferably red wine) per day is fine, but avoid other alcoholic drinks, especially cocktails, which are typically loaded with sugar.

- Soft Drinks: Sodas, including diet soft drinks should be avoided. As discussed in the *Lifestyles* and *Healthy-Gut* chapters, soft drinks wreak havoc on our health and have no place in an anti-aging program. As discussed in previous chapters, sweeteners should be omitted from the diet. People who consume artificial sweeteners are twice as likely to get diabetes as non-consumers. Sweeteners also create all kinds of problematic issues with gut bacteria.

- Fruit Juices: Should be eliminated from the diet, even freshly squeezed juices. Without the fiber to slow digestion and absorption of the sugars in them, they become concentrated sugar drinks that spike blood sugar.

Snacks

Healthy snacks may curtail mid-late morning and mid-afternoon, between meal cravings and hunger. They can also be eaten in place of a meal if you are on the run.

- Two hard-boiled eggs with salt and pepper to season.
- Hand full of almonds, walnuts, Brazil, or Macadamia nuts.
- Handful of grass-fed beef, bison, or venison.
- Chopped raw vegetables with guacamole, goat cheese, tapenade, or nut butter.
- Sauerkraut, pickles, or kimchee.
- Hummus with carrot and celery sticks.

- One sliced apple with one tablespoon almond butter.
- One serving of whole, low-sugar fruit such as berries, avocado (yes, avocados are considered fruit), grapefruit, orange, cantaloupe, apple, pear, kiwi, plum, peach, nectarine. You may spread a few tablespoons of almond butter on an apple or pear or have a few nuts with it.
- Grass-fed yogurt with ¼ cup of berries.
- Glass of grass-fed kefir.
- *Noggin Nosh* - Brain Ripening Superfood Nutrition Bar.
- Cup of bone broth.
- Half an avocado drizzled with olive oil, salt, and pepper.
- Sliced smoked salmon or lox with a spread of ricotta or cream cheese.
- Celery with cream cheese, almond butter, or cottage cheese.
- Canned tuna or sardines.
- Olives and nuts.
- Grass-fed cheese.
- Two squares of dark chocolate (70% cocoa and above) dipped in 1 tablespoon almond butter.

Treats/Desserts

Once your body has adapted to the new way of eating, cravings for sweet things and junk food will wane. That said, you may still want a treat now and then.

Some treats are actually good for you in moderation. Dark chocolate and red wine are not only delicious, but they are also rich in polyphenols (phytochemicals found abundantly in certain natural plant food sources that have antioxidant properties). I think of red wine and dark chocolate as healthy indulgences and have them both a few times per week. That said, don't overdo it. Stick with the one-two glasses of wine and have a few squares of chocolate (organic, 70% and above cocoa content) not more than once per day. I find with the latter a few squares are more than enough and I just cannot eat more.

It's okay to indulge in dessert once in a while, especially to celebrate a special occasion. I may share dessert at a good restaurant after consuming a meal of good quality fats and protein as that slows the digestion and absorption of the sugar. I especially like to eat dessert as a treat when in Europe as they typically don't over sugar desserts. European bakers tend to use top quality fats like grass-fed cream and butter, which has more nutrient content and as fats, will slow the digestion and absorption of sugar. The US tendency is to overuse sugar in almost every food product. We just don't have it right, and I'm not sure we ever did. America did give birth to the 'big food' companies.

If you choose to order a dessert once in a while, select the least sweet option and a dish that has plenty of fats in it like cream and butter, and only after dinner. I know this might seem counter-intuitive but eating dessert after a protein, fat rich dinner and a dessert rich in fat from butter and cream will actually reduce its impact on your body. The pancreas has a break processing the good fats and protein from the meal, and you will not experience an insulin spike. Remember, dessert is an infrequent option and totally a personal choice. It should not be a daily routine; it should commemorate a special occasion and enjoyed as a celebration.

If you are compelled to have dessert regularly, stick to basics like two squares of dark chocolate dipped in 1 tablespoon almond butter, a sliced apple dipped in almond butter, or a half a cup of berries topped with a drizzle of fresh, grass-fed, unsweetened cream.

Another little tip about treats, try to eat the healthiest options at least 80% of the time and 20% of the time you can indulge in treats and some of the foods not recommended in my program. This routine may be easier to transition to and will still yield great benefits. If you can manage a 90%-10% ratio that is even better. I have found going from a typical Western diet to my recommended plan may be a little tough for some people, so knowing you can have treats and go off the plan a bit makes confirmation easier.

*Cooking Methods

- Sautéing: Is the cooking method preferred over frying. Food should be prepared at low/med heat, never on high. Use grass-fed butter, extra virgin olive oil, virgin cold pressed, or unrefined coconut oil and add in white wine, fresh lemon juice, garlic, and herbs and spices to season. This is my preferred cooking method, and I use it several times a week to cook eggs, salmon, chicken breasts, and vegetables.

- Oven roasting or broiling: This cooking method can be used for chicken or meat but avoid oven roasting or broiling fish because the high heat damages the delicate omega 3 fatty acids. Baste chicken or meat with extra virgin olive oil or grass-fed butter, mustard, wine, balsamic vinegar, apple cider vinegar, fresh lemon juice, fresh prepared sauces or dressings, garlic, ginger, herbs, and spices.

- Baking: Meatloaf, chicken, steaks, or fish may be baked with broths or sauces of your choosing as immediately above. I choose to cook my organic dark-orange sweet potatoes this way and then add grass-fed butter to them after.

- Grilling on coals or lava rocks with gas: Grilling provides a great way to cook steaks, chicken, or fish. Make sure the cooking temperature it is not too hot with fish as it can damage the delicate omega 3 fatty acids. Baste whatever protein you choose with extra virgin olive oil or grass-fed butter, mustard, wine, balsamic vinegar, apple cider vinegar, fresh lemon juice, fresh made sauces or dressings, garlic, ginger, herbs, and spices.

- Boiling: I limit boiling to hard-boiled eggs. Boiling vegetables removes most of the nutrients from them.

- Steaming: This is a good way to cook vegetables. I typically drizzle extra virgin olive oil on steamed vegetables and fresh lemon and garlic, salt, and pepper to season.

- Stir-frying: I do not use the stir-fry method of cooking often. When I "stir-fry" it is actually more like sautéing as I don't cook anything at high temperatures.

Fast Food

- Superfood Smoothies: I drink a lot of smoothies and carry them in a small insulated cooler bag every day as I am out running around. If I know I will be out the entire day I will prepare two smoothies and pack to go with me. Smoothies are a great meal-on-the-go, a good snack options, or fantastic post-gym workout as well. One of my favorite things about these superfood smoothies is their nutritional value. They provide key macro and micro nutrients for folks on the go. I love to say; "*superfoods smoothies - better skin from within.*"

So what's in a "Superfood Smoothie?

I always start my superfood smoothies with filtered water or unsweetened almond milk. I occasionally use kefir as the base as well. Typically, I add a small handful of nuts or 2 tablespoons of almond butter, a portion of berries (alternatively an apple or pear), half of an avocado, a scoop of unflavored, unsweetened whey or collagen protein, a few stocks of broccoli, and a few stuffed handfuls of dark leafy greens such as kale, spinach, chard, or collard greens. I mix it up in an electric blender.

Play with your own formulas and see what you like. Don't use more than one portion of fruit however, as you will overdo the sugar. Buy some shaker bottles for storage and enjoy. Superfood smoothies are the best fast food I know!

Other Fast Food Options

- Grass-fed yogurt with blueberries and a handful of almonds.
- An apple, or orange with a handful of nuts.
- *Noggin Nosh* - Brain Ripening Superfood Bar.
- If you are desperate and have forgotten to bring the above recommended items, most fast food outlets can prepare a low-carb burger/sandwich by wrapping the protein (chicken, turkey, or beef patty) in lettuce. Make sure you tell them to hold sauces like BBQ or ketchup as they are loaded with sugar. Do not be tempted to add fries or a soft drink. Ask them for free water or buy bottled water.

Tips

- Be careful buying processed sauces and dressings as many of them contain added sugar and high omega 6 vegetable oils. It is best to make these items at home. They are not only much better for you - they are super easy to make as well. If you must purchase packaged products, read the labels. Try to find alternatives without added sugars or high omega 6 vegetable oils. For products that contain oil, make sure to buy them produced with extra virgin olive oil instead of other types of vegetable oils.
- Cook at home as much as possible.
- Use extra virgin olive oil for salad dressings. Use lower sugar balsamic vinegar, apple cider vinegar or fresh lemon juice (best option). Season with fresh garlic, mustard, herbs, and spices.
- Use natural salts such as Himalayan or Real Salt.
- Richly colored spices like turmeric, cinnamon, and cayenne are very healthy. They are rich in micronutrients like antioxidants. Use richly colored spices liberally in food preparations.
- Cut down on Omega 6 foods as they cause inflammation. As discussed, a typical Western diet is about 25:1 ratio of Omega 6 foods versus Omega 3 foods. In a perfect world, we should be at a 1:1

ratio. If you reach a 2:1 ratio or even a 3:1 ratio the overall diet will still yield good results.

- Protein portion size should be about the size of your fist or a deck of cards for each meal.
- Eat plenty of low-carb vegetables. Ideally, we want to keep your carb consumption around 100g/day. Read more about carbohydrates and fat loss in the *Weight Loss* chapter.
- The superfood smoothies may serve as meal replacements.
- Eat organic, pasture or free-range chicken only.
- Eat pasture eggs or organic omega 3.
- Eat grass-fed meats.
- Eat organic vegetables and fruits only.
- Use only extra virgin cold pressed olive oil, preferably organic.
- Use only virgin cold pressed unrefined coconut oil.
- Consume organic grass-fed, whole milk, yogurt, and kefir products.
- Eat and or cook with grass-fed butter.
- Eat grass-fed cheese.
- If you use cream or half & half, only use organic grass-fed.
- Eat at least one-two probiotic foods per day.
- Eat organic raw nuts and no-sugar-added nut butters.
- Starchy tuber vegetables – eat yams and/or dark orange or purple sweet potatoes.
- No regular potatoes, rice, or pasta.
- Empty your pantry/cupboards of all unhealthy temptations; chips, candy, ice cream, sodas, juices, bread, pasta, rice, cereals and baking ingredients like wheat flour, and sugar.

Times to Eat

Try to complete daily eating by 7 PM, or finish meals at least 3 hours before sleeping. Ideally, you should adopt a peak fasting schedule of 13-18 hours from the last meal (dinner) until breakfast and then wait 6-11 hours between meals each day. This meal routine provides many wonderful health benefits, which I write about more broadly in the *Intermittent Fasting* chapter.

Eating at Restaurants

- Do not eat bread.
- Do not request starch dishes on the side. Ask servers for substitute vegetable options instead. Most restaurants offer broccoli/broccolini, spinach, green beans, or asparagus as options and typically at no additional charge. You can have vegetables with butter, garlic, or lemon juice and they taste great!
- Make sure fish options are wild caught and request a wine-butter, lemon-butter, or garlic-butter sauce -- NO sweet sauces or garnishes.
- If you order beef ask for a burgundy sauce or wine-butter, lemon-butter, or garlic butter sauce -- NO sweet sauces or garnishes.
- Lamb or chicken should be prepared in the same manner -- NO sweet sauces or garnishes.
- Vegetables with butter, garlic, or lemon juice are fine and they taste great!

Happy Eating!

4

Exercise = Life Extension
(Secret 2)

"We do not stop exercising because we grow old; we grow old because we stop exercising."

~ **DR. KENNETH COOPER**

For many, exercise is a foul, cringe-worthy word. Shudder the thought of getting, up, out and moving! I don't know if it is laziness, a lack of knowledge of the importance, or just the failure to care for oneself; whatever it is, it is concerning because the benefits of exercise are immense and the consequences of being inactive dire.

A U.S. government study, completed in 2011, estimates that nearly 80 percent of adult Americans do not get the recommended amounts of exercise each week, potentially setting themselves up for years of health problems. Researchers at the Centers for Disease Control and Prevention (CDC) analyzed survey data collected from more than 450,000 U.S. adults ages 18 and older. The survey asked, "How often do you engage in physical activity outside of your job and for how long?"(1)

The recommended amount of exercise for adults, based on U.S. government recommendations, is a minimum of 2.5 hours of moderate-intensity aerobic exercise each week or one hour and 15 minutes of vigorous-intensity activity, or a combination of both as well as muscle-strengthening activities at least twice per week.

This recommendation is the base of how much exercise people should be getting, and if 80% of Americans are not even getting that, it presents a scary scenario!

It's important to remember that we evolved from nomadic ancestors who spent all their time moving around in search of food and shelter, traveling great distances on a daily basis. Although our survival no longer depends on these activities, the fact is our bodies were designed for movement and designed to be regularly active, not sitting around all day.

When physical activity diminishes as is typical with aging, the body sends signals (cytokines) telling the muscles to degenerate and organs to atrophy. Their function decreases because they have no reason to remain efficient. Inactivity will accelerate the aging process to the extent that it becomes a greater risk factor than simply growing older. A person who is not physically fit experiences lower bone-density, less lung capacity (the quantity of air you can exchange on each breath), and compromised stroke volume (the amount of blood your heart pumps with each beat) than a person in a physically fit condition.

Cytokines are messenger molecules that turn on or off metabolic pathways in the body's tissues and cells. Cytokine-6 (C6) is the master chemical for inflammation (think decay) and Cytokine -10 (C10) is the master chemical for repair and growth (think renewal). Exercise signals the body to produce C10, which triggers specific types of hormones and growth factors that induce repair, growth and renewal. Sedentary people produce excessive amounts of C6, which triggers perpetuate inflammation, prompts toxicity and radical decay.

Without exercise, you miss out on the body's precise internal ability to signal cells to act younger, which makes you look and feel younger. It is a continuum, the more you move, the less you decay.

Many experts agree as much as 70% of the body's decay may be forestalled until the "end." Don't think of exercise as work, think of it as 'grow' messages to your body. One of those messages is to reprogram your genes, to get leaner, stronger, and younger. The habits and routines of regular exercise lead to success.

REASONS TO EXERCISE

Regular exercise burns extra calories and makes your body more efficient at burning fat. As a result, your daily metabolism will be significantly higher. Exercise also stimulates the heart and reduces the risk of developing heart disease by as much as half. It strengthens bones and prevents osteoporosis; a condition affecting about one-third of adult women and 15% of men. Regular exercise also makes you feel good! Ever notice how exercise puts you in a good mood? It's not just your imagination. It produces a "natural high," stimulating the brain to produce hormones called endorphins, natural mood enhancers and painkillers.

Studies associate exercise with decreased symptoms of depression and anxiety, the most common psychiatric conditions affecting millions of individuals in the United States. Physical activity has consistently been shown to improve physical health, life satisfaction, cognitive functioning, and psychological well-being. Conversely, physical inactivity contributes to the development of psychological disorders. Specific research supports the use of exercise as a treatment for depression. Exercise compares favorably to antidepressant medications as a first-line treatment for mild to moderate depression and is documented to improve depressive symptoms when used as an adjunct to medications. (2)

Aerobic exercise increases the body's capillary network (blood vessels that supply the muscle cells with fuel and oxygen), muscle mitochondria, and stroke volume of the heart (more blood pumped with each beat). It improves the lung's oxygen delivery and boosts immune function by stimulating beneficial hormone flow. Exercise supports a more efficient circulatory system; strengthens bones, joints, and connective tissue so you can absorb increasing stress loads without breaking down. It boosts energy levels and leaves participants increasingly energized and refreshed, rather than slightly fatigued and depleted from more intense workouts.

Exercise delivers oxygen and nutrients to your tissues and helps the cardiovascular system work more efficiently. When the heart and lung health improves, you have more energy to for the rest of your daily tasks. Increasing physical activity helps control weight by preventing excess weight gain. Controlling excess weight gain keeps blood sugar levels balanced and regulates appetite.

When you engage in physical activity, you burn calories. The more intense the activity, the more calories burned. Low-level aerobic exercise trains your body to efficiently utilize free fatty acids for fuel, a benefit that is realized 24 hours a day, with a higher metabolic rate and a preference for fat over glucose. Exercise also increases circulation, which helps prevent erectile dysfunction and impotence and can increase sex hormones like testosterone in men. (3)

Brain Health

Scientific evidence based on neuroimaging approaches over the last decade has demonstrated the efficacy of physical activity improving cognitive health across the human lifespan. Aerobic fitness spares age-related loss of brain tissue during aging and enhances functional aspects of higher order regions involved in the control of cognition. More active individuals are capable of allocating greater attentional resources toward the environment and can process information more quickly. (4)

In a study conducted at the University of British Columbia, researchers found that regular aerobic exercise, the kind that gets your heart and your sweat glands pumping, appears to boost the size of the hippocampus, the brain area involved in verbal memory and learning.(5) Additional new research indicates exercise can keep cognitive ability sharp into old age and might help prevent Alzheimer's disease along with other mental disorders that accompany aging. (6, 7)

Disease Prevention

Physical inactivity is a modifiable risk factor for cardiovascular disease and a widening variety of other chronic illness, including diabetes, cancer (colon and breast), obesity, hypertension, bone and joint diseases (osteoporosis and osteoarthritis), and depression.

Several studies show incontrovertible evidence that regular physical activity contributes to the primary and secondary prevention of several chronic diseases including stroke, metabolic syndrome, type 2 diabetes, depression, some types of cancer, arthritis, falls, and may reduce the risk of premature death. There is a direct relation between the volume of physical activity and health status, such that the most physically active people are at the lowest risk. Interestingly, the greatest improvements in health status occur when participants who are least fit become physically active. (8, 9, 10, 11)

Anti-Aging

New research is hinting that exercise may have a more profound effect on the aging process than scientists were previously willing to believe. In 2007, Simon Melov Ph.D., Professor and member of the founding faculty at the Buck Institute for Research on Aging,* was part of a team that found that exercise appeared to reverse the effects of aging in a group of older Canadians. The study examined two groups of people, one older and one younger. The researchers took muscle biopsies from each participant, a painful procedure involving a long needle, and analyzed the "gene expression" patterns in the tissues—which genes were turned on and off. (Over time, different genes activate in various cells of the body, a process called "epigenetic" change). They then placed half of each group on a strict but not-too-demanding resistance exercise program for six months.

At the end of the six-month course, they took more biopsies and found the older subjects' muscles reverted to a "younger" state—that is, they had many of the same genes activated as their younger study mates. "We showed you could essentially reverse the gene expression signature of aging with exercise," wrote Melov.

In short, physical activity switched the "young" genes on, and the "old" genes off. Most of those genes had to do with the function of mitochondria, which can be considered the power generators of the cell, converting oxygen and nutrients into adenosine triphosphate (ATP). ATP is the chemical energy "currency" of the cell that powers the cell's metabolic activities. Mitochondria also take part in cell signaling and help cells sense and adapt to their environment. (12)

*The Buck Institute, based in Novato, California, is the nation's first independent research facility focused solely on understanding the connection between aging and chronic disease. Our mission is to increase the healthy years of life.

Mark Tarnopolsky, MD, Ph.D., professor and division head of Neuromuscular and Neurometabolic Disorders in the Department of Pediatrics at McMaster University, Hamilton, Ontario worked as Melov's coauthor. Dr. Tarnopolsky became fascinated by mitochondria and the role it played in the original study, so he continued from where the 2007 study left off.

Tarnopolsky's research focused on mitochondrial aging in mice, and he used genetically modified mice that had been programmed to undergo mutations to their mitochondrial DNA at a much greater rate than normal, which caused their mitochondria to wear out faster—which, in turn, made them age more rapidly. He then placed some of those mice on a regular treadmill exercise program, forty-five minutes, three times a week, while letting others stay sedentary in their cages.

The results were dramatic. The sedentary mice prematurely aged. They became gray, emaciated, and feeble. The mice that exercised were still healthy, active, and sported shiny black fur; they literally walked all over their sedentary cousins, despite the fact that they had the same broken mitochondrial DNA. The effects were far more than superficial. Autopsies showed the physically active mice had stronger hearts, healthier livers, brains, and robust reproductive organs compared to the inactive mice. Exercise had somehow repaired their mitochondrial DNA—in short; it reversed their aging. Tarnopolsky suspects exercise causes the mitochondria to transmit signals ordering molecules to repair other organs, not just muscle. (13)

Younger DNA

Additional new research has also shown that exercise can help keep DNA healthy and young. Anabelle Decottignies, Professor at the de Duve Institute at the Catholic University of Louvain in Brussels, and her colleagues found that just moderate-intensity physical activity helps hold back cell aging.

The team studied the designated part of DNA that keeps track of how many times a cell has divided. Each time a cell divides, it copies its

DNA (packed into chromosomes) and this section of the chromosomes, called telomeres, gets shorter. In the study, Decottignies identified a molecule responsible for directing this telomere-shortening. Until this work, scientist understood little about how the chromosomes controlled this DNA-snipping process. Decottignies recruited ten healthy people to ride stationary bicycles for 45 minutes and took a muscle biopsy from each of their legs before and after the cycling session. She also measured blood levels of muscle function with lactate; the cells muscles produce when stressed.

Based on analysis of the samples, researchers found that a compound called nuclear respiratory factor 1 (NRF1) protects the telomeres from being snipped away. They also documented exercise boosts NRF1. "Think about NRF1 like varnish on nails," says Decottignies. "You cannot change the nail, but you can change the varnish again and again. What you're doing is refreshing and replacing the old section with new protective molecules at the telomeres."

Decottignies explains the protection to the telomeres is refreshed with each bout of moderate exercise, thus helping the DNA, and in turn, the cells, to remain "younger" and hold off the aging process. "The protection is constantly renewed upon exercise," says Decottignies. (14)

THE HEALTHY HABIT OF EXERCISE

I'm sure you are thinking *do I have to?* Don't panic. Try not to see exercise as a daunting, painful task forced upon you. Think of it as a life changing, life-extending, fun new hobby. Something to make you feel fantastic, and reap incredible rewards!

You do not have to spend money, time at a gym, or on pricey equipment if you choose not to. You can easily create fun, simple routines at home using natural body exercises such as walking, running/sprinting, pushups, pullups, lunges, squats, plyometrics, even jumping jacks. You can also buy inexpensive dumbbells at Amazon, Walmart, or a sports store for home use.

As an absolute bare minimum, plan to commit 15-20 minutes of low-intensity aerobic movement every day. Preferably, you should be getting a bit more, and your exercise routine should include cardio, strength-training, and flexibility exercises such as stretching, rolling, and yoga. Your cardio and strength-training should also include high-intensity interval training (HIIT) and low-intensity sustained state (LISS) variations. Ensure that you get some form of exercise at least six days each week. I would suggest alternating cardio and strength exercise days such as:

- Monday: 45-minute strength training session, including 15 minutes of HIIT.
- Tuesday: 30-45 minute walk.
- Wednesday: 30-minute intense strength training session.
- Thursday: 30-45 minute stationary bike session.
- Friday: 30-minute intense strength training session with 3-5, 15-60 second treadmill, outdoor, or cycle sprints.
- Saturday: 30-45 minute brisk walk, hike, or session on elliptical or rowing machine.
- Sunday: Rest.

The example exercise program is purely for suggestion. There are many options and variations to incorporate into your routine. Plan to change things up frequently and intensify the workout depending on your fitness level. Do not let your body grow accustomed to a set routine so the more you switch it up, the better.

Once you choose the exercise(s) you want to do, plan how to fit the routine into your life. Establish a set time for exercise much like you would for an appointment. Plan at least 30- minutes for each workout. A good period to exercise is first thing in the morning, get it out of the way and free up the rest of the day. If morning doesn't fit into your schedule, try planning it in over your lunch hour or after work. A brisk walk after dinner is always good.

Before starting any exercise make sure to stretch and warm up. Warming the muscles improves the blood flow and reduces the risk of injury. Stretching is also important as it enhances flexibility and prepares the muscles for physical activity.

STRENGTH TRAINING

I like to mix strength training workouts and typically alternate a pushing exercise (push-up or triceps dip) with a pulling exercise (pull-up or bicep curl) in succession to create a high-intensity interval training workout.

Best strength training results come from a sporadic routine of varied workouts that are brief and intense. These exercises stimulate the release of adaptive hormones, such as testosterone and human growth hormone, helping improve body composition and delaying the aging process.

Strength training signals muscle growth and increased coordination as fine muscle detail through the elaborate networks of nerves that link the brain and the body. Weight training reverses nerve decay apparent with aging. It also brings neural connection out of hibernation by utilizing signal pathways. The signals have always been there; we just fail to use them.

Your routine should focus on exercises that engage a variety of muscles. I personally prefer doing real-life movements such as squats, pull-ups, and push-ups, instead of working isolated body parts with gym machines. That said, I do mix it up and use weights in the gym regularly.

Strength workout should be done three times per week on non-consecutive days and include upper-body pushing, upper-body pulling, lower-body, and core.

Exercise Examples:

- Upper-body pushing: Push-ups (regular, elevated feet, elevated hands), dumbbell chest presses, dumbbell shoulder presses.
- Upper-body pulling: Pull-ups, body-weight row, dumbbell row, rubber-band row, TRX row.
- Lower-body: Squats, lunges, step-ups, plyometric jumps/leaps.
- Core: Plank, supine march, push-up hold with leg lift, stability ball pike.

Exercise Directions:

Upper-Body Pushing Exercises

- Push-Up:

  1. Get into a high plank position and place your hands firmly on the ground, directly under shoulders.
  2. Tighten and squeeze your abdominals—as if you were about to be punched in the gut—and squeeze your glutes. Maintain these contractions for the duration of the exercise.
  3. Lower your body - keep back flat and eyes focused about three feet in front of you. Keep a neutral neck—until your chest grazes the floor.
  4. Pause at the bottom, and then push yourself back to the starting position as quickly as possible.
  5. Inhale on the way down, and exhale on the way back up.

- Elevated Hands Push-Up:

  1. Place hands on an elevated surface—such a box or bench—with your arms straight and your hands directly below your shoulders.

2. Walk your legs out behind you until you're in a pushup position. Your body should form a straight line from your head to your heels.

3. Tighten and squeeze your abdominals—as if you were about to be punched in the gut—and squeeze your glutes. Maintain these contractions for the duration of the exercise.

4. Lower your body until your chest nearly touches the box or bench. Don't let your hips sag at any point.

5. Pause at the bottom, and then push yourself back to the starting position as quickly as possible.

- Elevated Feet Push-Up:

1. Lie on the floor face down and place your hands about 36 inches apart from each other holding your torso up at arms-length.

2. Place your toes on top of an elevated surface (bench, bar stool, etc.). This position will allow your body to be elevated. (the higher the elevation of the feet, the higher the resistance of the exercise).

3. Tighten and squeeze your abdominals—as if you were about to be punched in the gut—and squeeze your glutes. Maintain these contractions for the duration of the exercise.

4. Lower yourself until your chest almost touches the floor as you inhale. Press your upper body back up to the starting position and exhale on the way back up.

5. Pause at the bottom, and then push yourself back to the starting position as quickly as possible.

- Dumbbell Chest Press:

1. Lie on the bench with a dumbbell in each hand and your feet flat on the floor.

2. Tighten and squeeze your abdominals—as if you were about to be punched in the gut—and squeeze your glutes. Maintain these contractions for the duration of the exercise.

3. Push the dumbbells up so that your arms are directly over your shoulders and your palms are up.

4. Lower the dumbbells down and a little to the side until your elbows are slightly below your shoulders, inhaling while doing so.

5. Roll your shoulder blades back and down, like you're pinching them together and accentuating your chest.

6. Push the weights back up, taking care not to lock your elbows or allow your shoulder blades to rise off the bench, exhaling while doing so.

- Dumbbell Shoulder Press:

1. Hold a dumbbell in each hand and sit on a bench with back support.

2. Plant your feet firmly on the floor about hip-width apart.

3. Tighten and squeeze your abdominals—as if you were about to be punched in the gut—and squeeze your glutes. Maintain these contractions for the duration of the exercise.

4. Bend your elbows and raise your upper arms to shoulder height, so the dumbbells are at ear level.

5. Place the back of your head against the pad.

6. Push the dumbbells up and in until the ends of the dumbbells touch lightly, directly over your head, exhaling while doing so.

7. Lower the dumbbells back to ear level, inhaling while doing so.

Upper-Body Pulling Exercises

- Self-Assisted Pull Up:

1. Place a chair, bench, or box beneath a chin-up station at a park, gym, or using a home chin-up bar. The chin-up bar should be high

enough so that when you stand on the chair, bench, or box and grasp the bar, your arms are slightly bent.

2. Place your hands on the bar using an underhand grip with your palms facing you.
3. Jump upward and pull yourself up with your arms until your chin clears the bar. Hold this position for a one-count, the slowly lower yourself back down.
4. Try to keep your abs tightened throughout the exercise.

- Regular Pull-Up:

1. Perform the exercise as above but without the assistance of the chair, bench, or box.
2. You can also try this with an overhand grip, with your hands facing away from you.
3. Allow your arms to extend fully between reps.

- Bodyweight Row:

1. Grab onto a bar in front of or above you with your hands shoulder-width apart.
2. Try to keep your abs tightened throughout the exercise.
3. Start with arms fully extended into a relaxed/hanging position.
4. Pull yourself up towards the bar and tuck in your elbows about 45 degrees from your armpits. Lead with your chest until your sternum touches the bar.
5. Lower yourself until your arms are fully extended again and repeat for the desired number of reps.

- Dumbbell Row:

1. Stand to the right of your weight bench, holding a dumbbell in your right hand with your palm facing in.

2. Place your left knee and your left hand on top of the bench for support. Let your right arm hang down and a bit forward.
3. Pull your abdominals in and bend forward from the hips so that your back is naturally arched and roughly parallel to the floor, and your right knee is slightly bent.
4. Tilt your chin toward your chest so that your neck is in line with the rest of your spine.
5. Pull your right arm up until your elbow is pointing to the ceiling, your upper arm is parallel to the floor, and your hand comes to the outside of the ribcage.
6. Lower the weight slowly back down.

- Rubber-Resistance Band Row:

1. Choose a resistance band based on your ability. The color-coded bands offer a variety of resistance levels; the lighter the color, the less resistance, and the darker the color, the greater the resistance.
2. Fasten the center of the resistance band to a stable piece of equipment or furniture. If a sturdy structure is not available, anchor the band by wrapping it around the center of your feet. Sit tall on the floor with your legs outstretched in front of you, knees slightly bent. Pull your abdominal muscles in toward your lower back and slide your shoulder blades down and away from your ears.
3. Hold an end of the band in each hand with an overhand grip. Turn your palms to face each other and extend your arms straight to assume the starting position.
4. Pull the handles toward you as your elbows bend and move slightly behind your torso. Keep your arms close to the sides of your body. Maintain a straight torso and avoid leaning forward or backward.

5. Stop pulling when your hands reach your body. Hold the contraction for one count, then straighten your arms to return to starting position.

Lower Body Exercises

- Squat:

  1. Place your feet approximately shoulder-width apart, bending your knees with a straight or slightly arched back.
  2. Always engage your core – squeeze and tighten your abs.
  3. Lower your torso all the way down until your butt is nearly touching the ground or least parallel to your legs.
  4. Your torso is between your knees, and arms extended in front. Start with body squats and add in dumbbell or barbell squats for a more intense workout and as your body adapts to the squats.

- Static Lunge:

  1. Keep your upper body straight, with your shoulders back and relaxed and chin up (pick a point to stare at in front -- don't keep looking down).
  2. Always engage your core – squeeze and tighten your abs.
  3. Step forward with one leg, lowering your hips bending both knees at about a 90-degree angle. Make sure your front knee is directly above your ankle, not pushed out too far, and make sure your other knee doesn't touch the floor.
  4. Position weight in your heels as you push back up to the starting position.
  5. To reduce the intensity of the exercise, hold onto a chair or other kind of support. If you want a harder workout, hold dumbbells at your side. Try to do 10 to 15 reps per side.

- Dynamic Lunge:

  1. Stand with both feet together and with your right leg take a long step forward.
  2. Always engage your core – squeeze and tighten your abs.
  3. Bend the back leg moving the knee towards the floor; the front knee should not go further forward beyond your toes.
  4. Your back knee should go down to an inch off the floor but not touch.
  5. In one controlled movement, return your front foot back to the starting position with the other foot.

- Step-Up:

  1. Before starting, find a step, chair, box, or bench to place your foot on.
  2. Place the right foot on the elevated platform.
  3. Squeeze and tighten your abs.
  4. Step on the platform by extending the hip and the knee of your right leg. Use the heel mainly to lift the rest of your body up and place the foot of the left leg on the platform as well. Exhale on the way up.
  5. Step down with the left leg by flexing the hip and knee of the right leg as you inhale. Return to the original standing position by placing the right foot to next to the left foot in the initial position.
  6. Repeat with the right leg for the recommended amount of reps and then perform the same exercise with the left leg.

- Plyometric Jump/Leap:

  1. Get into a squat position with your feet about shoulder-width apart.
  2. Squeeze and tighten your abs.

3. Squat and explode up using your entire body, including your arms.
4. Land softly on the balls of your feet.
5. Repeat in quick succession.
6. To increase workout intensity, use a box to jump on and add dumbbells.

Core Exercises

- Plank:

    1. Get into pushup position on the floor.
    2. Now bend your elbows 90 degrees and rest your weight on your forearms.
    3. Tighten and squeeze your abs and glutes (buttocks muscles).
    4. Keep your entire body straight and do not allow your midsection to sag.
    5. Hold for 20-30 seconds.
    6. For an advanced workout, extend one arm straight out in front, keep the weight of your upper body on the arm positioned on the floor. Alternate sides.

- Supine March:

    1. Lie on your back with your legs bent, your feet flat on the floor, and your arms on the floor with palms down.
    2. Draw your right knee toward your chest and simultaneously push your left knee into the floor, lifting your pelvis as high as you can.
    3. Contract your left glute for a one-count, lower your pelvis, and then repeat on the opposite side.
    4. Continue alternating sides until you have completed the number of reps on each side.

- Knee Fold Tuck:

  1. Sit tall, hands on floor, knees bent, squeezing a playground or workout ball between them.
  2. Lift knees, so shins are about parallel to the floor and extend arms.
  3. Pull knees toward shoulders, keeping upper body still. Bring knees back to starting position.

- Mountain Climber:

  1. From the push-up position, draw your right knee quickly towards your chest and then return it to the starting position and then follow with the left knee.
  2. Alternate sides as fast as you can until you achieved the desired reps.

- Stir-the-Pot Plank:

  1. Get yourself into a plank position and then rest your elbows on a large workout ball. Arms should bend at a 90-degree angle, and the entire body should form a straight line from head to ankles.
  2. Maintain a neutral neck position. Squeeze and tighten abs and glutes. Do not allow your head to move up or down, do not allow your hips to drop or your knees to bend, and make sure the your upper back does not round over by ensuring that your scapula is kept down and back at all times.
  3. From this position, move your forearms in a small circular motion while keeping the rest of the body stationary.
  4. After completing a full clockwise movement, perform the same movement counterclockwise.
  5. Continue until achieving optimal repetitions.

Notes

- Try to do 2-4 sets of each exercise and 10-15 reps per set.
- The described exercises may be considered a starting point and examples to build on. Intensify any of them based on your fitness level, and constantly change things up. Do not let your body get accustomed to anything so the more you switch the program up the better.
- Confused about technique? Google the exercise; there are numerous examples available online, both in video and text formats.
- Workout intensity should be aligned with energy and motivation levels. Push as hard as you can when you feel like it, and a bit lighter when you don't. That said, any exercise should require some level of effort.
- Turning up the intensity and rapidly doing the routines in succession can turn an ordinary workout into a high-intensity interval training workout (HIIT), which is highly recommended at least once a week, twice is even better!
- High-intensity, short-duration workouts stimulate the release of adaptive hormones—particularly testosterone and human growth hormone—contributing to a lean, energetic, and youthful body. Work hard and complete your session in less than an hour, even (or especially) if you are an experienced lifter. That's right—go against the Conventional Wisdom of long, drawn-out sessions of the same old sets using the same weight and repetitions. A 30 to 45-minute session is more than sufficient for most people.

CARDIO TRAINING

Low-intensity sustained state (LISS) cardio workouts should be done at least three times per week, and you can schedule them however you choose. They should also be done at 50 to 70 percent of your maximum heart rate and plan for between two to five hours per week total. Vary workout type, frequency, intensity, duration, and always align with energy levels.

High-intensity interval training (HIIT) cardio workouts should be done 1-2 times per week, and at 75 to 85 percent of your maximum heart rate.

Cardio Examples:

- Treadmill Walking: The advantage of treadmill walking is it is an indoor activity, therefore; you can exercise in any weather condition. You can also read, listen to music or watch TV to pass the time. Most computerized treadmills allow users to program an optimal training heart rate. The added programming makes it easier to control the intensity of your workout. The disadvantage of a treadmill is the investment of buying one for home use or the cost of joining a gym.

- Outdoor Walking/Running: Walking or running outdoors is a nearly perfect exercise. It requires nothing but a good pair of walking shoes and ideally a monitoring device to measure speed and distance. It is easy, free, and being outdoors on a beautiful day can send your spirit soaring. Weather conditions may make walking outdoors a disadvantage.

- Stationary Cycling: Stationary cycling is another great exercise. It is another indoor activity for any weather. Riding a stationary bike offers the luxury of reading or watching TV to pass the time. It is a good exercise alternative for people with knee or foot problems as it spares the joints. Most stationary bikes offer computerized programs to monitor training heart rates. The disadvantage is, you have to purchase a stationary bike for home use or join a gym.

- Outdoor Cycling: Cycling outdoors can be exhilarating, and a beautiful day this activity can lift your spirits. You obviously need to have access to a bike, and you should have a monitoring device to measure speed, time, and distance. It is also recommended to wear a helmet, as a safety precaution.

- Swimming: Swimming is an excellent activity for people suffering from arthritis or overweight. The buoyancy of the water reduces stress on joints and bones. Swimming at a brisk pace delivers a great cardiovascular workout, it burns fat and strengthens nearly all muscle groups.

- Rowing, Stair-Climber, or Elliptical Machines: Equipment generated exercises can be enjoyed indoors and in any weather. The disadvantages of exercise machines are cost and space in the home or the expense of a gym membership.

HIIT Cardio

- Sprinting: Sprinting can be done using any of the above exercises. You should do between 3-8 sets with all-out effort, lasting 15 to 60 seconds, depending on your fitness level. Rest for 45-60 seconds between each set. Total workout duration should be 10-20 minutes.

- Station to Station: Use any combination of exercises such as push-ups, pullups, lunges, squats, and jumping jacks. Depending on your fitness level, complete 3-8 sets with all-out effort, 10-15 reps per exercise, lasting approximately 15 to 60 seconds each. Rest for 45-60 seconds between each set. Total workout duration should be 10-20 minutes.

Notes

- Try to do regular cardio exercises for at least 30-45 minutes at a time.
- Sprints and station to station can also be combined.
- Make sure to include HIIT cardio at least once per week, ideally twice.
- Short, intense sprints trigger optimal hormone balance, lean muscle development, accelerated fat metabolism, and incredible fitness breakthroughs.
- Age is not an issue. Whether you are 20 or 75, you can find a form of sprint workout that suits you.

ESTABLISHING YOUR TRAINING HEART RATE

Determine your maximum heart rate by subtracting your age from 220. (Example: If you are 45 subtract that from 220, and you get 175 beats per minute)

Calculate your resting heart rate by counting your heart beats per minute when you are at rest, such as first thing in the morning. It's usually somewhere between 60 and 100 beats per minute for the average adult.

Calculate your heart rate reserve (HRR) by subtracting your resting heart rate from your maximum heart rate. (Example: if your resting heart rate is 80, subtract this from 175, which would give you a 95 HRR).

Multiply your HRR by 0.5 (50 percent). Add your resting heart rate to this number. (Example: 95 x 0.7 = 47.50 + 80 = 127.5)

The above in only an example and this particular example infers the low exercise intensity heart rate should be at approximately 127.5 beats per minute and their max high exercise intensity heart rate should be at 160.75.

It is also important to note the recommendations are a guide. You may have a higher or lower maximum heart rate, sometimes by as much as 15 to 20 beats per minute. If you want a more definitive range, consider discussing your target heart rate zone with an exercise physiologist or a personal trainer.

Keep track of your heart rate. The easiest way is to wear a sports smart band (available online or at a sports store). You may also monitor heart rate manually by taking your pulse. To take your pulse place two fingers on the side of your neck at the carotid artery or on the inside wrist. You should feel the blood pulsing through the artery. Count the number of beats or pulses felt in a 10-second interval. Multiply the number by 6 to determine the heartbeat per minute. (Example: if you count 20 beats in ten seconds x 6 = 120. Your heartbeat per minute is 120).

OTHER EXERCISES

Abdominals

Using correct form, most of the examples of exercises incorporate the abs. Adding crunches or leg lifts etc. to the routine is fine, but if you do so, make to practice them correctly. I throw a few sets of leg lifts while hanging from a pull-up bar at the gym several times per week, but I also engage my abs with almost everything else I do, including, walking, cycling, push-ups, and yes, even sitting.

When you are doing exercises such as push-ups, tighten your abs (pressing the navel toward the spine) and squeeze throughout the number of reps you are doing and repeat for the next set/s. Do the same while doing pull-ups, squats, lunges, curls, and any other exercise.

When engaged in daily movements such as walking, doing household chores, yard work, carrying kids, toting groceries, or driving practice tightening your belly muscles. Pretend someone is about to punch you in the gut while you blow out the candles on your birthday cake. Hold the contraction for 10, 20, or more seconds a few times every hour. To mix it up, squeeze your abs while slightly tilted to one side and then repeat on the other side.

Try to engage your abs in almost everything you do, and you will soon notice improved core muscle tone and a strong, functional set of abs will help you avoid back problems and perform activities more safely. Squeezing your abs is effective, and once you have done it for a while, it just becomes automatic, meaning you don't even think about it, you just find yourself doing it all the time.

Foam Rolling

One of my favorite things to incorporate into my workout is foam rolling. Foam rolling is a type of self-myofascial release in which pressure is applied to certain body parts to relieve pain. Once, a unique technique used only by athletes, coaches, therapists, and trainers it is now transformed into a common practice for people at all levels of fitness. Broader awareness, technology, and affordable products have introduced an increasing array of training and recovery methods. A recent study published in the Journal of Sports Rehabilitation found that foam rolling significantly increases the individual's range of motion and the combination of static stretching and foam rolling led to the greatest flexibility improvements.

I often warm-up and cool-down with foam rolling. I use it as therapy for stiff, sore muscles and joints, and also as a stress relief mechanism. I typically will use foam rolling for nearly every muscle group working from 30 seconds to several minutes in each area.

Lying face down and with the roller under my thighs I roll my quadriceps; alternating raising each leg I roll my abductors. Turning on my side,

I roll by IT bands; then, sitting on the roller, I roll my glutes. Allowing the roller to move further down I roll my hamstrings, then calves. Moving it up past the glutes to my lower back (this is my favorite area, and I spend a lot of extra time here) I roll here up and down for at least several minutes. I work my upper back and shoulder blades, the area I roll last and least is my stomach and chest area.

Stretching

You may think of stretching as a waste of time or a procedure designed for runners or gymnasts, but stretching is important for us delivers profound benefits. Stretching improves mobility and keeps muscles flexible, strong, and healthy, and we need that flexibility to maintain a range of motion in the joints. Without flexibility, the muscles shorten and become tight. When required to perform, weak muscles are unable to extend properly. That puts you at risk for injury, joint pain, strains, and muscle damage.

Think about sitting in a chair all day, do you notice how your lower back gets sore and hamstrings tighten? When this occurs, it makes it harder to extend your leg or straighten the knee all the way, inhibiting walking and reducing your mobility. Likewise, when tight muscles are suddenly called on for a strenuous activity involving running or jumping, they are damaged from sudden stretching. Injured muscles may become too weak to support the joints, which can lead to joint injury. Regular stretching keeps muscles long, lean, and flexible.

Basic stretching routines and additional options are featured on many online information sites.

Tips

- Regardless of your current physical condition, you can get fit in as little as a few hours a week. Commit to exercise regularly and strategically. Plan balanced routines that include extensive low-intensity movement, periodic high-intensity, short-duration strength-training sessions, and occasional all-out sprints.

- Warm up: Whatever exercise you choose on any given day, make sure to start by warming your body and muscles by walking slowly, cycling, or stretching, etc. to get blood out of your organs and moving to your muscles.

- Cool down: Make sure to wind down slowly -- never abruptly stop any activity. Winding down gives your heart and muscles a chance to return to normal, and prevents a sudden drop in blood pressure that can make you feel faint.

- Hydrate: Make sure to drink water while exercising and at least a glass after finishing.

- Limitations: If you have an orthopedic injury or other health condition be sure to ask your doctor which exercise is best for you.

- Avoids: Avoid consistent workout type, frequency, and intensity and be sure to alter your routine frequently, not only to account for your improved fitness level but to enjoy the psychological and physical benefits of evolving fitness goals and interests.

Avoid a repetitive schedule of sustained cardio workouts at medium to high intensity (above 75 percent of max heart rate). Occasional sustained harder efforts are okay.

Avoid prolonged strength training workouts conducted too frequently like hour-plus sessions of isolation exercise sets on any given muscle group.

Avoid excuses to not exercise. Consistency and commitment are critical to success.

MOTIVATIONAL QUOTES

"Use it or lose it."

"Sitting has become the smoking of our generation."

"We do not stop exercising because we grow old; we grow old because we stop exercising."

~ DR. KENNETH COOPER

"Those who think they have not time for bodily exercise will sooner or later have to find time for illness."

~ EDWARD STANLEY

"The desire of activity is designed by nature to promote our physical well-being. Physical activity is the law of physical health."

~ EDWARD BROOKS

"Lack of activity destroys the good condition of every human being, while movement and methodical physical exercise save it and preserve it."

~ PLATO

"Movement is a medicine for creating change in a person's physical, emotional, and mental states."

~ CAROL WELCH

"To keep the body in good health is a duty... otherwise, we shall not be able to keep our mind strong and clear."

~ BUDDHA

"You don't get the ass you want by sitting on it."

~ UNKNOWN

"Making excuses burns zero calories per hour."

~ UNKNOWN

"The hardest lift of all is lifting your butt off the couch."

~ UNKNOWN

5

In Need of Supplements?
(Secret 3)

"No matter how much it gets abused, the body can restore balance. The first rule is to stop interfering with nature."

~ DEEPAK CHOPRA

The subject of dietary "supplements" is a tough one for me. I come from a vitamin, mineral, and nutraceutical background and was a huge proponent of the value of such supplements at one time. The compelling results of significant scientific studies designed to measure the effectiveness of nutritional supplements served to convert me from my advocacy. I now realize the use (or overuse) of dietary supplements is overall an absolute waste of money. There are a few beneficial exceptions which I will highlight in this chapter.

Studies show highly touted "anti-oxidant" supplements such as Vitamins C, A, E, and beta-carotene are not only costly and ineffective, they may actually be harmful to your health. Such additives affect toxicity levels and may hinder your body's ability to produce its natural antioxidants. (1)

In 2009, a German scientist named Michael Ristow and his colleagues added more documentation of the adverse effects of certain supplements with a simple, subversive experiment. Ristow's team recruited forty young people to participate in a regular physical workout program. The participants each exercised for more than ninety minutes, five days a week. Each participant in the study was given a pill once a day during the trial. Half the subjects received an antioxidant supplement with high doses of Vitamin C and Vitamin E, while the other half were administered a placebo pill.

Physical exertion sharply increases oxidative stress, at least in the short term. For years, scientists puzzled over this cause/effect, concluding that exercise is healthy despite the higher levels of reactive oxygen species (ROS) that it produces. And indeed, it is possible to exercise to excess, even to the point of causing actual physical damage. If a person lifts weights one day after a month of inactivity, he would most likely experience muscle soreness from the exertion. This reaction was thought to be in part relative to oxidative damage. So for decades, athletes subscribed to taking antioxidant supplements in an attempt to mitigate ensuing soreness caused by rigorous training.

Ristow's research findings turned the oxidative stress theory on its head. He subjected his young (hopefully well-paid) volunteers to excruciating muscle biopsies both before and after the training period. As expected, both groups showed evidence of oxidative stress in their muscles after training, but Ristow discovered the subjects who had taken the supplements benefited far less from their exercise program than the ones taking the placebo. If anything, the antioxidants seemed to have significantly diminished the benefits of the training.

Here's why:

Normally, our bodies produce natural antioxidants, powerful enzymes such as superoxide dismutase and catalase, which soak up the excess free radicals that exercise produces. The supplemental antioxidants appear to block these potent enzymes. "If you take antioxidants, you preclude your own antioxidant systems from being activated," Ristow explained. "Not only antioxidants but other repair enzymes."

In other words, by taking supplements, we allow native antioxidant defenses to grow weak and lazy, leaving us more vulnerable to damage from ROS. Adding a little bit of stress, like exercise, helps keep the body's antioxidant defenses in tune. We adapt to the stress and come out stronger (not to mention live longer). "This is why the benefits of exercise last so much longer than the exercise itself," Ristow concludes. The same principle applies to caloric restriction, which I will cover more in the *Intermittent Fasting Chapter*. (2, 3)

What about Resveratrol?

When David Sinclair's "Resveratrol-in-Fat-Mice" study made headline news the demand for resveratrol supplements rapidly grew. Despite the immense media focus it attracted, there have only been a handful of human clinical trials on resveratrol—versus several published clinical trials on mice. Most of the human studies involving resveratrol have been very small, with just a dozen or so subjects. Out of these small trials, few have reported significant positive effects. One of those positive effects reported was a slightly improved glucose tolerance in older pre-diabetic adults with use. A couple of other small studies have indicated small beneficial effects on cardiac function. Other trials found no effect on insulin sensitivity, or cognition, or on blood pressure and other parameters, even in obese patients.

Veteran health reporter Bill Gifford writes in his book *Spring Chicken:*

> The reason for these disappointing results may have to do with the way humans metabolize the stuff [resveratrol]. Even at very high doses, very little resveratrol actually makes it into our bloodstream, because our bodies think it is a poison, it gets annihilated in the liver.

Another concern is that not all supplements labeled as "resveratrol" actually contain any resveratrol, or if they do, very little. The omission on the label does not come as a surprise considering the entire supplement market is only marginally regulated by the FDA.

For the above reasons, I recommend not wasting your money on supplemental resveratrol, which is rather expensive. Resveratrol is easy to absorb naturally and with a high bioavailability form such as that from red wine, red grapes, aronia berries, blueberries, cocoa, dark chocolate, peanuts, and pistachios.

WHAT I RECOMMEND; THE ABSOLUTES!

Vitamin D

Among the hierarchy of super vitamins - Vitamin D ranks as the superhero of the legion. The family of compounds in the vitamin D entourage includes; vitamins D1, D2, and D3 (*Cholecalciferol*). Research indicates this vital nutrient impacts some 2,000 genes in the human body.

Vitamin D – a fat-soluble vitamin known as the "sunshine vitamin" -- is naturally produced in the skin as a direct result of exposure to ultraviolet (UV) radiation from the sun. The list of beneficial contributions Vitamin D distributes toward a body's whole health and welfare is extensive. Perhaps the most critical purpose is to regulate normal functioning of the immune system and regulate the absorption of calcium and phosphorous.

Adequate doses of Vitamin D are essential for the development of bones and teeth and to increase the ability to fight certain infections and disease. The body requires Vitamin D for life. As we age, failure to get sufficient amounts raises the potential for developing bone abnormalities like osteomalacia (soft bones) and osteoporosis (fragile bones). Deficiency of Vitamin D is linked to a substantially increased risk of dementia and Alzheimer's disease.

A huge factor in developing and sustaining the health of bones and the immune system, research studies indicate Vitamin D also possesses far-reaching effects on the entire body including the brain. It boosts immunity and combined with tryptophan and DHA/EPA it increases brain serotonin concentrations and helps prevent and ameliorate some of the symptoms associated with ASD without conventional side effects. Vitamin D is shown to regulate enzymes in the brain and cerebrospinal fluid. This function impacts the manufacturing of neurotransmitters and stimulates nerve growth. Vitamin D serves to protect neurons from the damaging effects of free radicals as it reduces inflammation.

Significant medical studies point to other primary benefits including Vitamin D's role in decreasing the risk of multiple sclerosis, reducing the chance of developing heart disease, combating depression, and even protecting against influenza. (4)

Vitamin D is more than a regular vitamin it is a steroid hormone. The responsibility of protecting the body from the damaging influence of free radicals and reducing inflammation is best supported by vitamin D's effective regulation of gut bacteria.

Studies conducted in 2010 provided evidence to support the interaction of gut bacteria with vitamin D receptors. The research showed vitamin D receptors indeed sent the message to the gut to increase activity or turn it down. (5)

The link between diminished levels of Vitamin D and the onset of dementia has been the subject of clinical studies for some time. A recent trial conducted by a team of specialists at the University of Exeter, United Kingdom investigated nearly 2,000 patients' cognition through repeated MRI examinations, surveys, annual assessment and medical history for six years. The study found older patients with low levels of Vitamin D experienced a 122% increased risk of dementia compared to patients with higher levels. The published results confirmed the relationship between Vitamin

D deficiency and the substantially increased risk for all-cause dementia and Alzheimer disease. (6)

Evidence from clinical trials supporting the benefits of Vitamin D continues to mount. The more compelling data points to a relationship between low levels of Vitamin D and the increased risk of type 1 Diabetes, muscle and bone pain, cancers of the breast, colon, prostate, ovaries, and lymphatic system, and a 70% increased risk for dementia and Alzheimer's disease in older people.

Health providers now encourage the use of Vitamin D supplements to lower blood pressure, reduce the risk of heart attack, and protect against life-threatening diseases like cancer.

Sources for Vitamin D:

Most human bodies can produce an ample amount of Vitamin D with just 10 to 20 minutes of the mid-day sun. Sounds simple! Lifestyle choices and environmental factors often impair the ability to get sufficient amounts of Vitamin D through sun exposure alone.

Some of the variables affecting the lack of UV delivery include

- Pollution
- Use of sunscreen
- Buildings and other obstructions that block the sun
- Skin pigmentation

Natural Vitamin D exists in only a few foods. Vitamin D rich food sources include:

- Eggs (yolks)
- Shrimp

- Salmon
- Sardines
- Herring
- Swordfish

It is challenging to obtain consistently adequate amounts of Vitamin D through food consumption and sun exposure alone. Therefore, this is one of the supplements I recommend strongly.

How much is enough? The medical community continues to debate optimal amounts of vitamin D for an individual's healthy functioning. The National Institute of Health (NIH) recommends a daily intake of:

- 600 International Units (IUs) for children and teens
- 600 IUs for Adults up to age 70
- 800 IUs for Adults over age 70

It should be noted there is a possibility of too much of a good thing. Excessive consumption (*hypervitaminosis*) of vitamin D can lead to over-calcification of bones, hardening of the blood vessels and subsequent damage to the liver, lungs, and heart. While toxicity is unlikely at an intake of less than 10,000 IUs daily, it may be a side-effect of use. Common symptoms of hypervitaminosis include loss of appetite, headaches, nausea, dry mouth, constipation, and diarrhea.

My recommendations for vitamin D supplementation is to take vitamin D3 (Cholecalciferol) only as Cholecalciferol is absorbed and utilized by the body better than any other type of vitamin D. Take between 2000-5000 IU per day in a soft gel, not tablets or capsules. I personally like Nature Wise or Viva Naturals soft gels, both available on Amazon and each product uses extra virgin olive oil for the base liquid; most other manufacturers use sunflower or soy oil.

Omega-3

As previously mentioned in *Nutritional Intake*, omega-3 fatty acids are essential fatty acids – meaning the human body cannot naturally produce them so we must either obtain them from our diet or take supplements. We also established that DHA and EPA are the most beneficial forms of omega-3 fatty acids as they are easily assimilated by the body and have numerous efficacies and benefits that include:

The ability to act as an anti-inflammatory makes DHA and EPA effective in the treatment and prevention of hundreds of medical conditions. They help support heart health as well as normal growth and development of the brain. DHA and EPA are widely documented as effective in the treatment of various types of cancer, arthritis, and infertility. Below are additional benefits:

- Brain Development: Our brains are made up of 20% DHA, which must be replenished regularly. DHA and EPA generate neuroprotective metabolites and in double-blind, randomized, controlled trials - increasing the amount of omega-3 in a diet can increase brain function and boost focus and memory in both children and adults. It is also now believed to help with the neurological and visual development of infants.

- Decrease in Depression: Increased amounts of omega-3 in a body can act as natural antidepressants, improve mood, and relieve some symptoms associated with bipolar disorder and other forms of chemical imbalance.

- Support Heart Health: Higher levels of omega-3 can reduce arterial inflammation and plaque build-up as well as lower excess levels of triglyceride in the bloodstream. High levels of triglyceride can cause heart disease.

- Dementia and Alzheimer's: Research shows that omega-3 can slow the progression of Alzheimer's disease as well as reduce the onset of dementia. The fatty acids are thought to slow memory loss as well.

- ADHD: DHA and EPA combinations have been shown to benefit therapy for attention-deficit/hyperactivity disorder (ADHD), autism, mood disorders, dyspraxia, and dyslexia. DHA and EPA are also linked to lower dementia, improved focus and memory, learning ability, and enhanced mental skills of these individuals.

- Inflammation: As established, long-term inflammation can contribute to almost every chronic Western disease known including heart disease and cancer. Omega-3 fatty acids can reduce the production of molecules and substances linked to inflammation, such as inflammatory eicosanoids and cytokines and studies have consistently shown a relationship between higher omega-3 intake and reduced inflammation.

- Good for Your Skin: DHA is a structural component of the skin and is responsible for the health of cell membranes, which make up a large part of the skin. Healthy cell membranes result in a soft, moist, supple and wrinkle-free skin. EPA also benefits the skin in several ways such as oil production and hydration/moisture retention of the skin which prevents signs of premature aging, and acne. Omega-3s protect your skin from sun damage as EPA helps block the release of substances that eat away at the collagen following exposure to UV rays.

- Improves Sleep: Low levels of omega-3 fatty acids are associated with sleep problems in children and obstructive sleep apnea in adults. Diminished levels of DHA are linked to lower levels of the hormone melatonin which helps you fall asleep. Studies in both children and adults have shown that supplementing with omega-3 increases the length and quality of sleep.

- Rheumatoid Arthritis: Joint stiffness and pain related to rheumatoid arthritis can be reduced and improved with increased omega-3 fatty acids because of their anti-inflammatory efficacies.

- Asthma: Omega-3 fatty acids may lower the incidence of inflammation in asthma sufferers making it easier for patients to maintain proper lung function and reducing the dependence on medications typically used for asthma control.

(7, 8, 9, 10, 11, 12, 13, 14, 15, 16, 17)

There are two types of fish oils; Triglyceride (TG) and Ethyl Ester (EE). There is a heated debate among industry experts regarding which oil is best. EE forms are cheaper to produce than TG, but the EE form is missing a glycerol backbone. The absence of the glycerol backbone means the free fatty acids must be reconverted into TGs before being transported in the blood, and our bodies are not that efficient at this. Therefore, the amount of actual absorbable omega-3 is lower in an EE form. Studies have shown that a much greater percentage of omega-3s were absorbed by patients taking TG fish oil versus the EE form. It is much more efficient for the body to get your DHA and EPA requirements from fatty cold water fish. If this method is not practical, high-quality triglyceride form fish oil or algal oil provide the best alternatives. (18)

The two brands of omega 3 supplements I trust most are Nordic Naturals (Ultimate Omega) for triglyceride fish oil and DSM's Life's DHA for algal oil. I would recommend 2000-5000mgs per day. Both brands are available in liquid or soft gel form.

Astaxanthin

I wrote earlier in this chapter about antioxidants being a waste of money. There is, however, one that is worth taking. Numerous clinical studies have been conducted, and many more are underway. The research is proving significant human benefits from astaxanthin supplementation.

What is astaxanthin? Astaxanthin is a naturally occurring carotenoid found primarily in marine organisms such as microalgae, salmon, trout, krill, shrimp, crayfish, and crustaceans. The microalgae Haematococcus Pluvialis is considered the richest source of astaxanthin.

Astaxanthin is a nutrient with unique cell membrane actions and diverse clinical benefits. This molecule neutralizes free radicals or other oxidants by either accepting or donating electrons without being destroyed or becoming a pro-oxidant in the process. Its linear, polar-nonpolar-polar molecular layout equips it to insert precisely into the membrane and span its entire width. In this position, astaxanthin can intercept reactive molecular species within the membrane's hydrophobic interior and along its hydrophilic boundaries.

The extensive studies on astaxanthin indicate diverse benefits as well as excellent safety, tolerability, and bioavailability. In double-blind, randomized controlled trials (RCTs), astaxanthin showed these values and efficacies:

- Lowers oxidative stress in overweight and obese subjects and smokers.
- Blocks oxidative DNA damage throughout the body.
- Highly effective anti-inflammatory.
- Boosts immunity in the tuberculin skin test.
- Lowers triglycerides and raised HDL-cholesterol.
- Improves blood flow in an experimental microcirculation model

- Improves memory and learning.
- Protects the mitochondria against endogenous oxygen radicals conserved their redox (antioxidant) capacity, and enhances energy production efficiency.
- Improves elasticity in the skin by strengthening the collagen layer.
- Reduces the size of wrinkles and improves skin texture.
- Revitalizes photo-aged skin by quenching oxidative stress in all skin layers.
- Boosts proliferation and differentiation of cultured nerve stem cells.
- Improves eye fatigue, capillary blood flow, visual acuity, and reduces inflammation of the ciliary muscle.
- Improves reproductive performance in men.
- Improves reflux symptoms in H. pylori patients.
- Improves muscle and recovery in athletes and regularly active individuals.
- Lowers C-reactive protein (CRP) and other inflammation biomarkers.
- Protects the skin from UVA-induced oxidative damage.

According to the study *Nishida et al., (2007)* "Astaxanthin is the most powerful antioxidant known to science." Herewith some of its attributes:

- 500 times stronger than Vitamin E.
- 560 times stronger than Green Tea Catechins.
- 800 times stronger than CoQ10.
- 3000 times stronger than Resveratrol.
- 6000 times stronger than Vitamin C. [19]

The significant power of astaxanthin comes from its unique structure that allows it to quench free radicals in the inner and outer layer of the cell membrane, unlike other antioxidants. [20, 21, 22, 23, 24, 25]

There are only two reputable manufacturers of astaxanthin. Nutrex and the brand I prefer AstaReal as it is the most studied brand of astaxanthin in the world. AstaReal's successful clinical studies validate its efficacies on; skin health, anti-aging, muscle endurance and recovery, eye health, cognitive performance and neurovascular protection. I recommend taking 12mg per day as indicated by the cited research for the best results for all of the above categories.

Collagen Hydrolysate

A little background on Collagen. Collagen is the main structural protein of the different connective tissues present in our bodies. The primary source of collagen is fibrous tissues such as tendons and ligaments. Collagen is also abundant in the cornea, cartilage, bones, blood vessels, the gut, and intervertebral discs.

The collagen family consists of 28 different proteins accounting for 25% - 35% of the total protein mass in mammals. It plays a pivotal role in the structure of several tissues such as skin and bones, providing rigidity and integrity.

Type I collagen is the most abundant type in the human body. It forms more than 90% of bone organic mass, and it is the major collagen of tendons, ligaments, cornea and many interstitial connective tissues. It is also the main component of human skin (80%) with collagen type III making up the remainder of skin's collagen (15%). The unique physical properties of collagen fibers confer structural integrity to the skin forming a dense network throughout the dermis. The main function of this system is to provide structural support to the epidermis. Also, collagen and elastin together form the extracellular matrix providing the skin with its structure, elasticity, and firmness.

Collagen is mainly produced by fibroblasts in the connective tissues. Numerous epithelial cells also make specific types of collagens. Fibroblasts are connective tissue cells in the dermis which is responsible for producing and organizing the collagen matrix. Fibroblast activation and proliferation can stimulate an increase of collagen production. This process slows as we age and we start experiencing skin deterioration. Lifestyle choices and environmental aggressors, excessive UV exposure, smoking, medications, alcohol, stress, and lack of sleep accelerate the aging process. All these elements influence the formation of wrinkles, pigmentation disorders, and changes in the skin's elasticity, tonicity, and roughness.

How Does Supplemental Collagen Factor?

When collagen supplements were first introduced to the consumer market, I dismissed them as another gimmick. My initial rationale considered collagen as a protein. When it enters the stomach, collagen is broken down before ever making it to the skin. Given that process, I figured the efficacies to be non-existent.

The capsule forms of collagen contributed to my skepticism. I felt there could only be minimal amounts of the amino acids and peptides ingested in a capsule to produce any potential efficacy.

Since the initial introduction of collagen capsules, there has been numerous clinical trials conducted. The published results of those studies provide clear evidence that specific forms/types of collagen supplementation produce significant benefits on skin properties. These efficacies include; improved skin hydration and skin elasticity, reduction of wrinkles, prevention of skin water loss, and improvements in skin tone and texture. The correct collagen supplemental regime may restore the homeostasis of macro and micronutrients and support the physiology of cells and tissues within the skin. The results of the most significant results were based on continued use. Improvements are largely documented between weeks 4-8 of use.

The type of supplemental collagen used made a difference in trial results. Clinical success was based on the use of hydrolyzed collagen or collagen hydrolysates (CH). The main reason for the difference involves the amount of small peptides with low molecular weight found in CH. These peptides make digestion easier, and it is efficiently assimilated, and distributed throughout the human body. When taken orally, CH reaches the small intestine where it is absorbed into the blood stream, both in the form of small collagen peptides and free amino acids.

Through the network of blood vessels, these collagen peptides and free amino acids are distributed in the human body, particularly to the dermis, where they have been proven to remain up to 14 days. In the dermis, CH has a dual action mechanism:

- Free amino acids provide building blocks for the formation of collagen and elastin fibers.
- Collagen oligopeptides act as ligands, binding to receptors present on the fibroblasts' membrane, stimulating the production of new collagen, elastin, and hyaluronic acid. (26, 27, 28, 29)

The product and brand of collagen I recommend is Collagen Hydrolysate by Great Lakes Gelatin. Buy it in powder form and add a scoop (2 tablespoons) to a smoothie, yogurt, kefir, milk, or water. This amount will give you an additional 11 grams of high- quality protein plus the collagen peptides and amino acids.

WHAT I RECOMMEND AS OPTIONAL

Whey Protein

Whey protein is worth taking to ensure getting enough daily protein in your diet. That said, if you follow my 'Nutritional Intake' plan, you should be getting adequate amounts. If you are short any specific day, incorporate collagen hydrolysate into your daily intake (see: benefits mentioned above). Collagen hydrolysate provides 11 grams of protein per serving. Days when you don't eat enough quality protein, and you don't want to double or triple up on collagen hydrolysate (it is a bit more expensive than whey), whey protein is worth keeping as a backup. It is a high quality, easily digestible protein containing all of the essential amino acids and it has numerous health benefits including:

- Increases fat loss while sparing lean muscle.
- Curbs hunger by creating a feeling of satiation.
- Enhances exercise recovery.
- Prevents muscle loss.
- Boosts immunity.
- Promotes healthy bone growth.
  (30, 31, 32, 33, 34, 35)

I only recommend unflavored/unsweetened whey protein concentrate (it tastes great on its own but can easily be mixed with fruit or into the types of smoothies I recommend in the 'Nutritional Intake' chapter) and preferably grass-fed. I personally use Jarrow and find it an excellent quality product and very well priced.

Creatine

I know you might find this surprising and think creatine? *Isn't that only for bodybuilders or athletes?* Creatine is a natural amino acid found in meat and fish, and small amounts are produced by the kidneys, pancreas, and liver. It plays an important role in releasing energy when an individual performs short-duration, high-intensity exercise and this energy significantly boosts muscular performance.

I include creatine as an 'optional' recommended supplement because it is one of the most researched supplements of all time with numerous proven benefits that include:

- Anti-aging properties.
- Brain and memory boosting.

- Muscle sparing.
- ATP (adenosine triphosphate) boosting properties (ATP is a chemical energy molecule produced in the mitochondria that your cells use to provide for their fuel needs).
- Helps overcome the effects of sleep deprivation and boosts mood state.
  (36, 37, 38, 39, 40, 41, 42, 43, 44).

Despite common myths promoted by the media, creatine is extremely safe and is used in certain clinical settings to treat neurological diseases. (45, 46)

The only creatine product I recommend is manufactured by the German company AlzChem AG. Their product, branded as Creapure is a patented form of creatine monohydrate and widely considered to be the purest and finest quality micronized creatine monohydrate commercially available today. AlzChem uses their proprietary manufacturing process to produce creatine monohydrate, ensuring it is free from impurities and unnecessary by-products including creatinine, dicyandiamide, dihydrotriazine, and thiourea.

Recommended usage: Men can take up to 1 teaspoon (5g) per day in water, or blended in a smoothie. Women should take ½ -1 teaspoon (2.5-5g) per day.

THINGS I DO NOT RECOMMEND

There are other substances out there that claim to have anti-aging benefits, such as Metformin, HGH (human growth hormone), testosterone, estrogen, and TA-65, etc. I have not seen clinical data validating efficacies on any of these substances and have searched extensively. I do not believe these materials provide significant, nutritional or health benefits, only the potential for harm. The only time any of these substances should be used is if prescribed for specific medical conditions that warrant their use.

- Metformin (a drug for treatment of type 2 diabetes): may have shown some potential anti-aging benefits in some circles, but the side effects far outweigh any potential positive effects.

- HGH (human growth hormone): Has been hyped and heavily promoted by A4M (The American Academy of Anti-Aging Medicine) with many of its anti-aging doctor members prescribing it - claiming there are numerous anti-aging benefits with plenty of supporting clinical studies proving its efficacies. There are ZERO such clinical trials proving the claims they make. So why do so many doctors specializing in anti-aging prescribe such products? Very simply, they recommend the supplements because those products are big profit generators with monthly treatments averaging $2000 per month.

I should add that I was a member of A4M and resigned after a year as I discovered the organization became too focused on pushing drug therapies and less concerned about promoting proven methods of age preservation such as those mentioned in this book. I subscribe the reasons for the industry philosophies are profit driven. Practitioners can make far more money from drug therapies than from sound, prudent advice that is often free.

HGH does have benefits for children who might suffer from stunted growth or dwarfism, but beyond those applications it should be left alone as it carries far too many health risks. Incidentally, the U.S. Food and Drug Administration (FDA) warns that taking HGH poses serious health risks, including being linked to an increased risk of cancer. (47)

- Testosterone/Estrogen: These are additional hormones promoted by A4M and its doctor members. Unless physician prescribed for a specific health condition, stay clear of these hormones as the side effects from use are just too great!

- TA-65 (its chemical name is cycloastragenol): A molecule isolated from various species in the genus astragalus and is PURPORTED to have telomerase activation activity). There have been many supplements claiming anti-aging benefits over the years with limited or no REAL clinical studies validating their claims. TA-65 is another such hyped supplement. TA-65 claims the ability to lengthen telomeres (protective caps at the end of DNA) - the length of telomeres is a marker of your biological age.

Scientists have discovered each time a cell divides, its telomeres get shorter, and when your telomeres get so short that the cell can no longer function, that cell either dies or enters into a permanent resting state called senescence. This discovery led researchers to investigate telomeres as a possible key to longevity. The theory held that if your telomeres can be restored to an earlier length, this will, in turn, lengthen your lifespan. This is the "scientific" angle TA-65 manufacturers promote to get your money!

6

Intermittent Fasting
(Secret 4)

"If you want something you've never had, you've got to do something you've never done."

~ THOMAS JEFFERSON

Fasting is nothing new. The practice has been around a very long time. I must admit, however, when I first heard of the 'miraculous' benefits of fasting a few decades ago, I was extremely skeptical. Since that time there have been extensive clinical studies conducted on intermittent fasting (IF). I have read and processed my share of the research findings, and the conclusions have eliminated my skepticism. I am not only a believer but a practicing advocate of several variations of intermittent fasting. I am totally sold on the benefits of IF, and it is now one of the pillars of my personal anti-aging regimen.

Numerous studies indicate IF can have profound and highly beneficial biological effects on the body and brain. IF appears to change the function of cells, genes, and hormones. The benefits this produces include: improved brain function, loss of body fat, lowered blood pressure, improved heart health, improved insulin sensitivity and glucose uptake – reducing Type 2 diabetes risks, decreased oxidative damage and inflammation, boosts cellular repair processes, may help prevent degenerative brain diseases and cancer, and may extend your lifespan.

Many other health benefits are achieved when individual genes are 'turned on.' Repair to specific tissues occurs that would not otherwise be altered in times of surplus. One could conclude that this genetic adaptation allows individual cells to live longer (as repaired cells) during famine because it's energetically less expensive to fix a cell than to divide and create a new one.

Brain Health

Dr. Mark Mattson, Chief of the Laboratory of Neurosciences at the National Institute on Aging Intramural Research Program in Bethesda, Maryland, and Professor of Neuroscience at Johns Hopkins University has conducted extensive research on the benefits of intermittent fasting.

In one study, Mattson and his colleagues found that intermittent fasting can help improve neural connections in the hippocampus while protecting neurons against the accumulation of amyloid plaques, a protein prevalent in people with Alzheimer's disease. "Fasting is a challenge to your brain, and we think that your brain reacts by activating adaptive stress responses that help it cope with disease," writes Mattson. He continues:

> From an evolutionary perspective, it makes sense your brain should be functioning well when you haven't been able to obtain food for a while. When you're hungry, your mind better be active and figuring out how to find food, how to compete and avoid hazards to get enough food to survive.

Additional research indicates fasting can significantly reduce the effects of aging on the brain. IF has potent anti-inflammatory effects on the entire body and many prominent scientists now believe that it is one of the key strategies for maximizing brain function. (1)

Dr. Mattson and his colleagues also discovered not only does IF improve physical health, but it also actually seems to be good for the brain. The study of mice (and later humans) fed on alternating schedules were found to have higher levels of brain-derived neurotrophic factor or BDNF. (2, 3, 4) BDNF levels govern the formation of new neurons and the development of synapses and various lines of communication within the brain. Higher levels of BDNF lead to healthier neurons and better communication processes between these neurological cells. (5) BDNF also helps stave off degenerative conditions like Alzheimer's and Parkinson's and helps preserve long-term memory. Low levels of BDNF are linked to dementia, Alzheimer's, memory loss, depression, and other brain processing problems (6, 7). It is important to note, BDNF decreases when our bodies are on a simple carb-high sugar diet. (8)

Alzheimer's disease is the world's most common neurodegenerative disease. There is currently no cure for the condition, so prevention is critical. In additional research studies, Mattson and his colleagues show that IF may delay the onset of Alzheimer's disease or reduce its severity (9). Intermittent fasting may also protect against other neurodegenerative diseases, including Parkinson's and Huntington's disease (10, 11), and shield the brain against damage due to strokes. (12)

Disease Prevention & Longevity

Dr. Valter Longo, biogerontologist, cell biologist, professor at the USC Davis School of Gerontology with a joint appointment in the Department of Biological Sciences, and director of the USC Longevity Institute has also conducted extensive research on the benefits of IF.

Longo initially studied fasting in mice. His early work showed that only two to five days of fasting each month reduced biomarkers for diabetes, cancer and heart disease and produced other significant health benefits. The research has since expanded to include humans, and scientists noted a similar reduction of disease risk factors. (13, 14)

Dr. Longo pointed out the health benefits of fasting may result from the fact that fasting lowers insulin and another hormone called insulin-like growth factor (IGF-1), which may be linked to cancer and diabetes. A reduction in these hormones may slow cell growth and development, which in turn helps slow the aging process and reduce risk factors for disease. "When you have low insulin and low IGF-1, the body goes into a state of maintenance, a state of standby," Dr. Longo said. "There is not a lot of push for cells to grow, and in general the cells enter a protected mode."

Longo ran additional studies to figure out why his starved yeast was living longer (15, 16) and what that might mean for humans. Why yeast? Yeast is one of the simplest eukaryotic organisms and many essential cellular processes are the same in yeast and humans. It is, therefore, an important organism to study to understand the initial molecular processes in humans.

As Bill Gifford writes in his book *Spring Chicken*:

> Longo discovered that at the deep cellular level, metabolism and longevity are so closely intertwined they are inseparable. These metabolic pathways all radiate from an essential cellular compound called mTOR (mechanistic target of rapamycin), which is perhaps best thought of as the main circuit breaker in a factory. When the breaker is switched on, the factory (that is, the cell) goes humming along, forging amino acids into the proteins that are the building blocks, messengers, and currency of life. When the breaker is off, the cell switches to a maintenance mode. It "recycles" old damaged proteins and by cranking up autophagy, cleans up the junk that accumulates in our cells over time.

Longo found that blocking the mTOR pathway caused his yeast to live three times longer. The result led him to believe that many of the effects of caloric restriction come about because the lack of nutrients compromises mTOR—an effect observed not only in yeast, but also in worms, flies, and mice. (Like the sirtuins, mTOR is conserved, meaning it appears up and down the tree of life.) Turning down mTOR also inhibits many of the growth pathways which seem to be connected with aging. With the mTOR breaker switched off, protein manufacturing is shut down, and cells don't divide as rapidly, so the animal does not grow. Instead, its cells become healthier. They also resist stress better, use fuel more efficiently—and thus are less susceptible to damage. It's a classic example of beneficial stress response, or hormesis (a biological phenomenon whereby a beneficial effect such as improved health, stress tolerance, growth or longevity, results from exposure to low doses of an agent that is otherwise toxic or lethal when given at higher doses). And it makes sense evolutionarily: When food is scarce, there is no point in wasting energy on growth.

Working with colleagues on additional research, Longo had an epiphany about his studies on yeast and the nature of cancer. When he starved the yeast, they not only lived longer, they became immensely resistant to stress of all kind, like oxidative stress caused by free radicals, and exposure to toxins. Meanwhile, although tumor cells seemed invincible, Longo knew that they were not. Cancer cells must eat perpetually, and in the typical body, loads of glucose is readily available for them to feast. Doctors can locate tumors by injecting them with glucose carrying a chemical tag. The tumors suck up all the glucose and then light up with the tag. Longo realized the nature of their glucose absorption made tumors potentially vulnerable. Because tumor cells were always eating, always growing, their mTOR was turned up exponentially — which reduced their stress resistance. In the lab, he demonstrated that subjecting cancer cells to added stress, by taking away their food, really did weaken them.

Longo proposed a radical experiment to his colleagues: He wanted to test mice with cancer and starve some of them for as long as they could tolerate it. He then blitzed the mice with massive doses of chemotherapy drugs, which are highly toxic to all cells.

The results of the experiment surprised everyone. In some of the trials, all the animals exposed to starvation before treatment survived the chemo, in contrast to all the regularly fed mice that died following chemo. The short-term fasting appeared to have switched the animals' healthy cells into a protected state, while the tumor cells remained more vulnerable to the chemotherapy agents. This "differential stress resistance," could make the drugs more effective by targeting them at the cancer cells themselves; the cancer cells would be unable to adapt, while the noncancerous cells were in a protected state because of the fasting so they would suffer less collateral damage. (17)

Longo and his colleagues eventually replicated the experiment on humans. Their first trial they found ten late-stage cancer patients who were willing to give it a try on a voluntary basis. The participants fasted for between two and five days in conjunction with a cycle of chemo. Surprisingly, all ten reported less severe side effects from the treatment after fasting. In some patients, the chemo also appeared to be more effective. (18)

The human trials represented only a small pilot study. The results were intriguing enough to prompt five larger clinical trials involving short-term fasting in conjunction with chemotherapy. Human studies consisting of about one hundred patients each are underway at USC, the Mayo Clinic, and in Leiden, the Netherlands, as well as a few other locations. Early results are certainly not conclusive but promising. Longo writes:

> The key mechanism, we think, is really what I call death by confusion. The idea is that normal cells have evolved to understand all kinds of environments, and cancer cells have de-evolved in some sense; they're very good at doing a few things but are just generally bad at adapting to different environments, especially if they are extreme.

Additional research by Longo and his colleagues showed that fasting rejuvenates the immune system and reduces cancer incidence in C57BL/6 mice, promotes hippocampal neurogenesis and improves cognitive performance in mice, and causes beneficial changes in risk factors of age-related diseases in humans (19).

Cynthia Kenyon Ph.D., a molecular biologist, and professor at the University of California, San Francisco, has conducted extensive research on the longevity of roundworms, specifically Caenorhabditis elegans or C. elegans as they are commonly called. Why test roundworms and how could research relating to the aging of humans?

Approximately 40% of C. elegans' genes are closely related to human genes. There are some human-like aging genes in the C. elegans that are connected to and affected by hormones insulin and IGF-1. Kenyon and her team were able to double the lifespan of the C. elegans by tweaking specific genes. As part of their research, the team also gave a batch of C. elegans sugar, and it shortened their lifespan by revving up the insulin pathway. Kenyon was so shocked by the results she immediately changed her own diet and eliminated sugars and most carbs. Her research has shown that controlling aging genes like insulin and IGF-1 will activate other genes that govern youthfulness and longevity. (20)

Heart & Overall Bodily Health

Researchers from the Intermountain Medical Center Heart Institute (IMCH) based in Salt Lake City, Utah conducted two separate studies on the benefits of intermittent fasting involving more than 200 participants (patients and volunteers) recruited at IMCH. Both studies resulted in positive results for overall health and heart health, but with the second study in particular, the researchers reported that fasting not only lowers one's risk of coronary artery disease and diabetes but also causes significant changes in a person's blood cholesterol levels. (21)

That discovery expands on the original IMCH study that revealed an association between fasting and a reduced risk of coronary heart disease, the leading cause of death among men and women in America. In the new research, fasting was found to reduce cardiac risk factors, such as triglycerides, weight, and blood sugar levels.

The researchers noticed that after 10 to 12 hours of fasting, the body enters into a self-protection mode and starts scavenging for other sources of energy throughout the body to sustain itself. Unlike the earlier research by the same team, the second study recorded reactions in the body's biological mechanisms during the fasting period. The participants' low-density lipoprotein cholesterol (LDL-C, the so-called "bad" cholesterol) and high-density lipoprotein cholesterol (HDL-C, the so-called "good" cholesterol) both increased (by 14 percent and 6 percent, respectively) raising their total cholesterol - and catching the researchers by surprise.

Dr. Benjamin D. Horne, Ph.D., MPH, director of cardiovascular and genetic epidemiology at the Intermountain Medical Center Heart Institute, and the study's principal investigator, said:

> Fasting causes hunger or stress. In response, the body releases more cholesterol, allowing it to utilize fat as a source of fuel, instead of glucose. This decreases the number of fat cells in the body. This is important because the fewer fat cells a body has, the less likely it will experience insulin resistance or diabetes.

The study also confirmed earlier findings regarding the effects of fasting on the human growth hormone (HGH), a metabolic protein produced by the pituitary gland to fuel growth and development in children. It also maintains some bodily functions, like tissue repair, skin homeostasis, muscle growth, brain function, energy, and metabolism, throughout life. During 24-hour fasting periods, HGH increased an average of 1,300 percent in women, and nearly 2,000 percent in men. Additional studies confirm the fasting related HGH increase. (22, 23)

Worth mentioning, the body naturally slows its production of HGH as we age, but high levels of insulin and IFG-1 production accelerates with aging. Higher levels of insulin and IFG-1 slows the body's ability to produce even reduced levels of HGH. When the body produces an insulin release after carbohydrate ingestion, HGH is inhibited. (24, 25)

HGH and insulin perform opposite functions in the body. HGH focuses on tissue repair, lean tissue (muscle) retention and growth, efficient fuel usage and anti-inflammatory immune activity. Insulin provides energy storage, cellular division, and pro-inflammatory immune activity.

Fat/Weight Loss

As discussed in the *Weight Loss* chapter, intermittent fasting facilitates fat loss. When you don't eat for a while, several things happen in your body. Your system initiates the necessary cellular repair processes and changes hormone levels to make stored body fat more accessible. These heightened biological functions lower insulin levels, produces higher growth hormone levels, and increase amounts of norepinephrine (noradrenaline). These associated actions boost the breakdown of body fat and facilitate its use for energy. (26) IF also increases your metabolic rate by 3.6% to 14%, helping you burn even more calories. (27, 28)

This process is contrary to what many people are taught. Conventional wisdom proposes that fasting lowers the metabolism and forces the body to hold on to fat in a so-called starvation mode. Reality is much to the contrary. Fasting supplies the body with benefits that can accelerate and enhance weight loss; specifically, fat loss. IF works on both sides of the calorie equation - it boosts your metabolic rate (increases calories out) and reduces the amount of food you eat (reduces calories in).

Type 2 Diabetes Prevention

Type 2 Diabetes has become far too common in recent decades. It is a devastating disease that is self-induced by poor dietary choices. The main characteristic of diabetes is high blood sugar levels in the context of insu-lin resistance. Anything that reduces insulin resistance should help lower blood sugar levels and protect against type 2 diabetes, and IF has shown to have significant benefits for insulin resistance and lead to the reduction of blood sugar levels. Clinical studies have shown that IF can reduce blood sugar levels and can reduce insulin levels by 20% to 31%. The research also suggests that IF may be highly protective for people who are at risk of developing type 2 diabetes. (29, 30)

Oxidative Stress & Inflammation Reparation and Prevention

We established that insulin and IGF-1 contribute to oxidative stress and inflammation which can cause premature aging and trigger other diseases. Oxidative stress helps create an environment promoting unstable mole-cules called free radicals, which react with other important molecules (like protein and DNA) and damage them. It is also determined that correct nutritional intake and IF may combat and potentially prevent the dam-age. Additional studies show that IF may enhance the body's resistance to oxidative stress as well as help fight inflammation, another key driver of all sorts of common diseases, as discussed in various chapters. (31, 32, 33)

Cellular Repair

IF stimulates the body's natural cellular repair processes as it triggers a metabolic pathway called autophagy (the processes by which your body removes waste material, cleans out various debris, including toxins, from cells, and recycles damaged cell components), signaling the body to reju-venate itself. (34)

INTERMITTENT FASTING METHODS

There are a variety of ways to fast. My suggestion is to figure which one you are most likely to maintain. I have tried all of the versions, and my favorite by far is 'peak fasting' also called time restricted feeding (TRF) or the 16:8 diet. Why is it my favorite? I have found it easier to adapt to and easier to manage. That does not mean it has to be the right method for everyone. It may be best to experiment a bit before settling on one protocol. Most successful programs end up incorporating a few different approaches on a routine basis. The most important thing is to bring IF into your life, embrace it, and realize the benefits are totally fantastic!

Peak Fasting

The methodology here is to fast every day by restricting your daily eating to a specific window of time. This process helps to move the body from burning sugars as a fuel source and on to burning fat, a far superior fuel source. As discussed in the *Weight Loss* chapter, results may take a few weeks. Each body must transition, but once the system has shifted over from burning sugar to burning fat as its primary fuel, you will find it easy to stay on this program. Fat is a slow-burning fuel. It allows the body to keep going without suffering from the dramatic energy crashes associated with sugar.

The eating window should be 8-10 hours and the fasting period should be 14-16 hours. For example, if you eat your last meal (dinner) at 7 pm, you would want to wait to eat your first meal between 9 and 11 am the next day. You may drink water and herbal tea during the fasting periods and add fresh lemon juice or a tablespoon of raw apple cider vinegar to these beverages as this boosts the body's cleansing function. Do not have any food for at least 3 hours before bed. Stick to the foods recommended in *Nutritional Intake*.

To kick-start the routine, and depending on your personal needs, the initial eating period could be 6 hours until your body is burning fat as fuel. Once this happens and you lose the weight you desire, add a few hours to the eating period to say 8-10 hours, which is kind of like a 'maintenance' stage.

The 5:2 Diet

This method is quite popular and recently made trendy by a few celebrities who reportedly used it to successfully lose weight.

The 5:2 diet involves eating normally five days of the week while restricting calories to 500-600 on two days of the week. On the fasting day, women should eat 500 calories, and men 600 calories. For example, you might regularly eat on all days except Mondays and Thursdays, where you eat two small meals (250 calories per meal for women, and 300 for men).

As with peak fasting, you may drink water, herbal tea, and you may add fresh lemon juice or a tablespoon of raw apple cider vinegar to either as this boost the body's cleansing function. Do not have any food for at least 3 hours before bed and stick to the foods recommended in *Nutritional Intake*.

Eat-Stop-Eat

Eat-Stop-Eat involves a 24-hour fast, either once or twice per week. An example, if you finish dinner on Monday at 7 pm, you would not eat again until dinner the next day at 7 pm. You can also fast from breakfast to breakfast, or from lunch to lunch. The result is the same.

If you are doing this to lose weight, then it is important to eat an average meal during the eating periods. Meaning, eat the same amount of food as if you hadn't been fasting at all.

The problem with this method is that a full 24-hour fast can be somewhat difficult for many people.

As with peak fasting, you may drink water, herbal tea, and you may add fresh lemon juice or a tablespoon of raw apple cider vinegar to either as this boost the body's cleansing function. Do not have any food for at least 3 hours before bed and stick to the foods recommended in *Nutritional Intake.*

Alternate-Day Fasting

Also, called the "every-other-day-diet," this method means you fast on one day, and then eat as you choose on the next day. This way you only need to restrict what you eat half of the time. On fasting days, you can drink as much water, herbal tea etc. as you like. Unsweetened and creamer free coffee and caffeinated tea are fine as well. As with the other fasting plans, stick to the foods recommended in *Nutritional Intake.*

HOW LONG DO YOU FAST?

IF can be continued until the desired weight loss is achieved or in perpetuity if you like its benefits and the way you feel. I have made it a permanent part of my lifestyle. Some days, such as when I am traveling, I go off, no big deal. Once your body goes into burning fat as opposed to carbs your body doesn't immediately switch back. Having the odd day off from it will have little effect.

7

Weight Loss

"There are risks and costs to action. But they are far less than the risks of inaction."

~ JOHN F. KENNEDY

Admittedly, I am not promoting a weight loss program. However, if you fully commit to this program, which includes correct nutritional intake, intermittent fasting, and exercise, weight loss, or specifically fat loss, is one of the many benefits your body will experience. Within a few weeks of starting the program, your body will begin using stored fat as energy. You may experience a loss of one to two pounds of body fat per week. You will physically transition from the very unhealthy, pro-inflammatory, fat-store 'merry-go-round' cycle, which not only keeps you overweight, but radically increases the risk for chronic diseases, AND ages you prematurely.

One of the goals and subsequent benefits of the program's nutritional intake is to put the body in a state of ketosis. What is ketosis? Ketosis is a condition in which the body is efficiently burning fat as its primary fuel source instead of glucose. By following my recommendations, you will convert your body from a sugar burner to a fat burner. The transformation is accomplished by reducing your consumption of carbohydrates, increasing the intake of fat, consuming an adequate amount of protein to meet your body's needs, and following an intermittent fasting schedule.

Simply restricting the amount of consumed glucose and starches will help your body naturally shift to preferring fat for fuel. Your cells automatically adjust their mechanisms to handle the increased levels of fat and lipid-based fuels. It takes a matter of weeks to reach that conversion, but once it's there, they are fairly robust transfers that don't just go away.

Consuming more fats and reducing carbs enhances the body's fat burning function. Enzymes are up-regulated and other metabolic processes are required to burn fat more efficiently, therefore making it easier for your body to tap into stored adipose tissue as an energy source. When your body reprograms gene expression to extract fuel from fat whenever it wants, hunger tends to subside, and blood sugar and energy levels stabilize.

Feeding the body a steady supply of carbs conditions it to burn glucose and keep the fat stores locked in. One of the several problems with this process is carbs do not burn as cleanly as fat, and they produce 30 to 40 percent more free radicals than fat. Free radicals damage important cellular structures, such as your mitochondrial DNA, cell membranes, and proteins like the mitochondrial electron transport chain. Carbs not only drive insulin levels up, but they increase the chances of becoming leptin resistant, which interferes with your ability to lose weight.

This plan does not represent another gimmicky low-carb fad diet – it is essentially a design of how humans were evolutionarily designed to eat. Many indigenous cultures, from the Inuits of North America to the Maasai of Africa, traditionally subsisted on diets consisting of macronutrient ratios very similar to ketogenic diets. These societies have thrived on this type of diet for thousands of years without the major health complications that plague most modern civilizations today.

So, how does a ketogenic diet work? Approximately 70% of the daily nutritional intake of a ketogenic diet should come from good fats I recommend, 25% from protein sources, and about 5% carbohydrates.

Don't panic about the reduced carbohydrates; there are still plenty of carbs in this diet, they are just concentrated in the right kinds of carbs. Ketogenic is not a low total carb diet, but a low, non-fiber carbohydrate diet. Limiting non-fiber carbs is a central aspect of the total ketogenic diet plan.

It is important to make the good carb/bad carb distinction. For example, vegetables are carbs, but they are fiber carbs. Fiber carbs will not push your metabolism in the wrong direction — only the non-fiber carbohydrates will (sugars and anything that converts to sugar, such as processed grains, pasta, rice, bread, cereal, cookies, and sugary drinks such). Calculate non-fiber carbs by subtracting the grams of fiber from the grams of total carbohydrate content in the food.

As a general guide, the level of non-fiber carbs that allows the body's entry into nutritional ketosis is on average about 50 grams per day or less of digestible or absorbable carbohydrates. However, we all vary how we respond to the same food, so this is not an exact recommendation. Some people, for example, can be in a full state of ketosis at a level of non-fiber carbs that's higher than 50 grams; maybe 70 or 80 grams. Other individuals, especially people who are insulin resistant or have type 2 diabetes, may require between 30 and 40 grams per day.

Incidentally, a diet rich in fiber has many additional health benefits. Among the benefits, fiber is highly valuable for the digestive system; it helps to keep bowel movements regular; the body uses fiber as a prebiotic for beneficial bacteria; and some of the fiber is converted to short chain fats to be burned as fuel for cells in place of sugar.

An additional note on fat and as set out in the *Nutritional Intake* chapter, quality fats include; avocados, olives, cacao butter, organic cold pressed coconut oil, extra virgin olive oil, omega 3 from wild fish or high quality triglyceride fish oil supplements, pasture eggs, grass-fed meats, organic grass-fed butter, almonds, walnuts, Brazil nuts, macadamia nuts, and organic nut butters, seeds such as black sesame, cumin, pumpkin and hemp seeds, MCT Oil, lard and tallow.

Do not include the fats found in the standard American diet. Omega-6 – polyunsaturated (PUFAs) oils and fats, wreak havoc on our health and to make matters worse, 85 to 90 percent of those oils are from genetically modified (GM) corn and soy.

Avoid all artificial sweeteners, none of them are safe, and they do not promote weight loss. As natural health expert, and author of *Fat for Fuel*, Dr. Joseph Mercola says:

> Artificial sweeteners, and most sugar alcohols with the exception of moderate amounts of xylitol, don't have calories, so they trick your body into thinking that it'll receive sugar (calories), but because the sugar doesn't arrive, the body ends up sending more signals, resulting in more carbohydrate cravings. This results in worsened insulin sensitivity and brain function, and increased risks for cardiovascular disease, stroke, and Alzheimer's disease are some of the severe effects of artificial sweeteners. Steer clear of products that contain aspartame in particular, as it's known to be the worst of all artificial sweeteners today.

Carb Consumption Overview

Listed are the approximate target carbohydrate amounts for daily consumption. Individual tolerance will vary. Through trial and error - you will find the levels that work best for your body. The recommended numbers are based on averages.

- 30 – 50 grams per day: Minimizes insulin production and maximizes fat metabolism. Within a few weeks of starting the program, your body will go into a state of ketosis, and you can lose up to two pounds of body fat per week. The weight loss includes the stubborn and dangerous visceral fat. I would advise you to start the program in this zone if you have body fat you need to lose.

- 50 - 100 grams per day: Will also minimize insulin production and will accelerate fat metabolism. You can lose one to one and a half pounds of body fat per week in this zone, and your body will stay in ketosis. This zone and the 'maintenance' zone are the best zones to stay in once you have lost the body fat you need to avoid the fat store "merry-go-round" cycle.

- 100 - 150 grams per day: Will keep you in a maintenance zone.

- 150 - 200 grams per day: Throws the body back in a fat store and weight gain mode as well as triggers the body to start producing too much insulin, the problems this cycle creates in described in previous chapters.

- 200 or more grams per day: Totally crosses the danger zone. This level of carbohydrate ingestion represents the typical American diet. Putting yourself here causes your body to over-produce insulin, store fat, and gain weight. Extended periods in this zone will wreak havoc on your health.

It is easy to drift into one of the threatening zones by adding grains, sodas, and sugary snacks back into your diet. To optimize total health and delay the effects of aging, dodge the carbohydrate trap. An occasional slip-up will not result in diet disaster, but try to stay disciplined here. Do not become vulnerable by eating one "bad snack" each day or even a few times a week.

TIPS AND CLOSING POINTS

- If there is no noticeable fat loss after a month to six weeks and you have been consistent in zone 1 or 2, reduce your carbohydrate intake even further.

- As discussed, minimizing carbohydrate intake controls insulin production and enables stored body fat to be burned for energy.

- Optimize fat intake to achieve high satiety levels, provide energy, and eliminate hunger.

- Optimize protein intake to preserve energy levels and maintain or increase lean muscle while you exercise.

- Fat loss is ramped up when you incorporate intermittent fasting (IF) into the diet regimen. I highly recommend IF to maximize anti-aging benefits and for overall health. After reading the IF chapter, you can determine the IF method that best fits your lifestyle.

- Many workout proponents believe they can eat what they want as long as they exercise heavily/regularly enough. The reality is no one can lose fat effectively with exercise-driven weight-loss efforts only. You MUST adjust eating habits along with exercise to moderate insulin production and convert your body from a sugar burner to a fat burner.

- The variable for your energy needs and total calorie consumption is fat. By committing to success, you make a concerted effort to eat just enough food to feel satisfied and energized. Since fat has a high satiety factor, a little goes a long way. A handful of nuts can sustain for hours if you skip a meal or need a quick bite to keep going. With the right meal choices and healthy snacks, your intensive weight-loss experience will not suffer the typical struggle and deprivation of a restrictive diet. Achieving the optimal body fat desired, you can begin to consume even more liberal amounts of fat without worrying about gaining weight.

- It's important to remember; it takes some time to convert your body from a state of burning sugar to burning fat as its primary energy source. The length of time will vary with each person, but the typical transition period can range anywhere from 3 to 6 weeks.

- When your body is in a state of ketosis, it starts producing ketones. Ketones are by-products of fatty acid catabolism (breakdown of fat) and can replace glucose as a primary fuel source for cells of the brain. The brain cannot directly utilize long-chain fatty acids for fuel since these types of fats cannot cross the blood-brain barrier. However; ketones can efficiently pass through the barrier, and your brain becomes more proficient at utilizing ketones over time. If you are interested in learning more on the subject, Dr. Emily Deans, board-certified psychiatrist and instructor at Harvard Medical School discusses the physiology of the efficiency of ketones work in the brain in an article published in *Psychology Today*. (1)

8

Healthy Gut - Healthy Brain
(Secret 5)

"A pessimist sees the difficulty in every opportunity; an optimist sees the opportunity in every difficulty."

~ WINSTON CHURCHILL

There is an old saying, "Always trust your gut!" That sage advice applies to many real-life situations, but there is a solid biological foundation in the guidance.

Research studies provide substantial, convincing evidence linking our guts to many health issues, including brain disorders. Lifestyle choice is considered by most the culprit contributing to our unhealthy microbiomes. So, what is a microbiome? The microbiome is defined as the collective microorganisms (100 trillion organisms - bacteria, bacteriophage, fungi, protozoa, and viruses) that live inside and on the human body. Our human microbiome is made up of communities of symbiotic, commensal and pathogenic bacteria which call the human body home. Their purpose is to perform life-sustaining functions that would be physically impossible without their support.

These communities exist in unique, complementary blends and inhabit everything from our skin and genitals to our mouths and eyes, and, of course -- our intestines. The clusters of bacteria from different regions of the body are variously known as microbiota including, for example, your skin microbiota, oral microbiota, vaginal microbiota and gut microbiota -- also known as gut flora.

The communities in our microbiome carry out a variety of functions which are vital to our health and well-being in fact, to our very survival. Microbiomes establish the parameters in which our bodies judge whether or not something is friend or foe. It maintains harmony, balance, and order amongst its communities, ensuring that opportunistic pathogens are contained to a minimum while keeping the host system from attacking itself.

It is our first, second and third line of defense – starting with the skin, through the mucus membranes, and finally the gut, providing a living barrier that can be modified and transformed to suit individual needs and unique environments.

Our gut microbiota is fundamental to the breakdown and absorption of nutrients. Without it, the majority of our food intake would not only be indigestible, but we would not be capable of extracting the critical nutritional compounds needed to function. Symbiotic cohorts not only provide this service but also secrete beneficial chemicals as a natural part of their metabolic cycle.

As infants we come into this world with a blank slate of sorts, awaiting the first contact with the microscopic organisms (microbes) surrounding us. The first exposure occurs in the birth canal, followed by a gut-nurturing infusion of mother's milk. The introduction is nature's way of establishing the foundation on which we will build our microbiome. These microbes play essential roles in the development of the human immune systems and once established, they provide energy sources and vitamins that we humans cannot manufacture on our own. They produce ingredients that act as anti-inflammatories and send signals to our brain. "Good" microbes help fend off the "bad" ones, and we cannot survive without them.

Familial, dietary, and environmental exposure throughout our developing years cultivates our ecosystem. The ecosystem serves an important role in the determination of our health for a lifetime.

As understanding of the microbiome's impact on our health grows, so does the realization that current bacteria-phobic trends must come to an end. It's time we cultivate a partnership with our microbiome.

Antibiotics and an obsession to sterilize our environments have resulted in a significant rise in gut-related illnesses. The escalation of disease serves to increase pressure on the medical community to invest resources to this area of human biology.

Research has uncovered an intricate web connecting gut flora to virtually every process in the body. As such, imbalances in the microbial communities are implicated in countless health issues including immune health, psychological well-being, and many other chronic health problems.

Research studies conducted at the California Institute of Technology published results adding significant findings to the growing evidence of microbiomes' influence on the brain. One study documented mice that became susceptible to autism-like symptoms as a result of infections suffered by their mothers during pregnancy also showed changes in their microbiomes. When researchers treated the animals with healthy gut bacteria, some of the abnormal behaviors and anxiety diminished. (1, 2)

Techniques and methods on how to manipulate one's microbiome have begun to flood medical literature. Trading gut bacteria are among the latest focus of therapeutic treatments, being successfully utilized as a means to treat antibiotic resistant infections. Some publications go so far as to suggest the therapy as a potential means of treating obesity.

Studies on the human microbiome are hailed as the new frontier of medicine. Prominent researcher scientists like Martin Blaser, professor of microbiology at the New York University School of Medicine and founder of the Foundation for Bacteriology, advocate good bacteria as "the new antibiotics."

SO WHAT IS CAUSING OUR MICROBIOMES TO BECOME INCREASINGLY UNBALANCED AND UNHEALTHY?

There are scientific indications the Western population's microbiome has changed in the last century and not for the better. A study led by researchers at the University of Oklahoma (3) focused on microbiome samples taken from ancient people, including Otzi the Iceman. Otzi lived around 3,300 BCE, his remains were found in the Otztal Alps. The results of the study support the hypothesis that ancient human gut microbiomes are more similar to those of non-human primates and rural non-western communities than to those of people living a modern lifestyle in the United States. From the data, the researchers concluded that the last 100 years represents a time of rapid change to the human gut microbiome, especially in cosmopolitan areas. Dietary changes, as well as the widespread adoption of various aseptic and antibiotic therapies have largely benefited modern humans, but many studies suggest the benefits come with a cost, such as the recent increase in autoimmune related risks and other health conditions.

Some of the culprits include:

- Processed foods: Containing high sugar concentrations and other chemicals.
- Chlorinated/chemically treated water effectively destroy intestinal microflora.
- Sugar: Studies suggest sugar can promote the growth of bad bacteria in the gut. This could lead to irritation in the gut, which could even manifest itself as an autoimmune response (allergies and skin

conditions are two milder problems). There's even recent evidence suggesting depression is actually your body's response to swelling in the gut. (4, 5).

- Overuse of antibiotics damages microflora.
- Artificial Sweeteners and Diet Sodas: Research studies involving mice showed consumption of artificial sweeteners altered the gut bacteria of mice in ways that made them vulnerable to insulin resistance and glucose intolerance — both of which can lead to weight gain. In other mice research published results report the association of artificial sweeteners and a drop in the appetite-regulating hormone leptin. Leptin is the hormone that inhibits hunger. (6)
- Increased exposure to powerful antibiotics and residues in foods also destroy intestinal microflora.
- Increased incidence of C-section deliveries deprive infants of exposure to vital microorganisms in the birth canal that "seed" the gut.
- Formula-fed babies show significant differences in their microbiomes compared to breastfed babies.
- Gluten: Dr. David Perlmutter writes in his books *Grain Brain and Brain Maker*:

While a small percentage of the population is highly sensitive to gluten and suffers from celiac disease, it is possible for virtually everyone to have a negative, albeit undetected, reaction. Gluten sensitivity—with or without the presence of celiac—increases the production of inflammatory cytokines, which are pivotal players in neurodegenerative conditions. *Gluten's 'sticky' attribute interferes with the breakdown and absorption of nutrients, which leads to poorly digested food that can then trigger the immune system, eventually resulting in an assault on the lining of the small intestine. Once this happens, the immune system sends out inflammatory chemicals in a bid to get things under control and neutralize the effects of the enemies. This process can damage tissues, leaving the walls of the intestine compromised (called 'leaky gut syndrome').*

Further to the above, according to Harvard's Dr. Alessio Fasano:

> Exposure to the gliadin protein (a protein found in gluten) in particular increases gut permeability in all of us. That's right; all humans have some degree of gluten sensitivity. Once you have a leaky gut, you're highly susceptible to other food sensitivities in the future. You're also vulnerable to the impact of LPS making its way into the bloodstream. Lipopolysaccharide, or LPS, is a structural component of many microbial cells in the gut. If LPS gets past those tight junctions, it increases systemic inflammation and irritates the immune system—a double strike that puts you at risk for a myriad of brain ailments, autoimmune disease, and cancer.

SO WHAT CAN BE DONE TO IMPROVE YOUR MICROBIOME?

For starters, you can improve your microbiome by reducing or eliminating a high carb, processed foods, genetically modified anything, sugar, and wheat rich diets. Other food products contributing to poor gut health are factory-farmed meats which come loaded with antibiotics. As the research indicates, consumption of carb-laden, processed, GMOs, sugars, glutens, and commercially grown foods change the gut bacteria for the worse. Rather than nourishing the body with life-enhancing, microbiome-supporting nutrients, these foods have the opposite effect. They introduce irritants, allergens, carcinogens, and inflammation into your body, thus setting you up for a variety of chronic illnesses.

Avoid taking antibiotics as much as possible. Antibiotics have a carpet-bombing effect on gut microbes. They indiscriminately take out everything in their path — including the productive gut flora your body needs to support long-term health. I understand in some cases, antibiotics are an absolute necessity, but they are way over-prescribed, overused, and represent a huge contributor to poor gut health.

Things that benefit your gut:

- Daily servings of cultured and fermented probiotic* rich foods such as; sauerkraut, kimchi, kombucha, pickled veggies, yogurt, and kefir encourage the growth of good bacteria. This subject will be discussed further in the *Nutritional Intake* chapter.

- Prebiotic foods: Non-digestible short-chain fatty acids that help your good. bacteria flourish such as artichokes, garlic, leeks, dandelion greens, beans, oats, onions, and asparagus.

- A diet that keeps blood sugar balanced also keeps gut bacteria balanced. A diet high in rich sources of fiber especially derived from whole fruits and vegetables feeds the good gut bacteria and produces the right balance of those short-chain fatty acids to keep the gut lining in check.

- Reducing gluten or avoiding it altogether will further improve gut health as well as healthy brain physiology.

- Research on calorie restriction and intermittent fasting has shown improvement in strains of good bacteria. One such study; (7) published in the specialty journal *Nature* in 2013, demonstrated calorie restriction enriches strains of bacteria that are associated with increased lifespan and reduces those strains that negatively correlate with lifespan. In the paper, researchers noted, "animals under calorie restriction can establish a structurally balanced architecture of gut microbiota that may exert a health benefit."

- Another great way to boost microbial exposure is simple; open the windows and let the microbes flow. Welcome them into your home, your car, your office – the more, the merrier, and the better for your microbiome. Move outside and get your hands dirty – as in; do some gardening! Plant flowers, mow the lawn, take a walk in the woods, participate in activities that connect you and your immune system with the trillions of microbes in the soil.

HEALTHY GUT = HEALTHY BRAIN?

Scientists have now determined that humans have two brains. The second brain is called the enteric nervous system. This brain resides in the gut. It is made up of groups of neurons living in the walls of the nine meters from your esophagus to your anus. It has more neurons than the spinal column or central nervous system, and in fact, the second brain contains a wide range of additional hormones and neurotransmitters, including ninety-five percent of the serotonin (the neurotransmitter associated with mood and some behaviors) in the body and fifty percent of the dopamine (a neurotransmitter associated with pleasure and the reward system) in the body. (8)

Long thought to be only concerned with directing digestive contractions, the enteric nervous system has an express conduit to the brain - the vagus nerve. Ninety percent of the vagus nerve consists of fibers dedicated to carrying communications from the gut to the brain. If you've ever experienced butterflies in your stomach from young love, excitement, anxiety, or felt like you knew something "in your gut," the sensation may have simply been your gut brain relaying messages to your brain, giving the adage 'gut instinct' real meaning.

Research thus far into the gut-brain relationship has suggested that probiotics* can have a positive effect on behavior, mental outlook (i.e., depression, anxiety), and brain function. One such study was conducted with a group of 36 healthy women who were divided into three groups. One group consumed yogurt containing probiotics for four weeks, one group ate yogurt without probiotics, and the remaining group was the control. After undergoing magnetic resonance imaging (MRI) of the brain and participating in emotion recognition tests, the researchers found the women who regularly ate yogurt with probiotics showed positive changes in brain function related to emotions and sensory processing. (9)

Understanding the relationship helps to clarify why the process of taking care of the gut and the brain within in it also helps improve the health of the brain in your head.

*Lactobacillus Plantarum (found in kimchi, sauerkraut, and other cultured vegetables) is one of the most beneficial bacteria in your body.

9

Sleep
(Secret 6)

"It is a common experience that a problem difficult at night is resolved in the morning after the committee of sleep has worked on it."

~ JOHN STEINBECK

Sleep is an integral part of optimizing the anti-aging process, and it works synergistically with all the other components of the program to deliver the best results possible.

Sleep plays a vital role in good health and well-being throughout your life. It is a fundamental, highly organized process regulated by complex systems of neuronal networks and neurotransmitters. Getting enough quality sleep at the right times can help protect your mental health, physical health, quality of life, and safety.

Sleep plays an imperative role in the regulation of the central nervous system and physiologic body functions, including cell renewal throughout the body, which is optimized during the evening restoration period. During sleep, the recovery and rejuvenation of muscles, organs, and all the systems of the body are accelerated. The restoration is guided by the sleep hormone melatonin, manufactured in the pineal gland (also dubbed the "third eye") near the center of the brain. This tiny organ regulates your daily and seasonal circadian rhythms, the sleep-wake patterns that determine your hormone levels, stress levels, and physical performance.

The circadian rhythm governs our sleeping and eating patterns as well as the precise timing of important hormone secretions, brain wave patterns, and cellular repair and regeneration based on a 24-hour cycle. When we interfere with our circadian rhythm we disrupt some of the very processes we depend upon to stay healthy, happy, productive, and focused.

Sleep was long thought to be a passive state, but we now understand sleep to be a dynamic process. The brain is active during sleep (but responding to internal stimuli, not external), and it drifts in and out of various sleep stages, or cycles. Our natural sleep pattern is to progress from light sleep (rapid eye movement [REM], when you dream and can be woken easily) into escalating stages of deeper sleep cycles (non-REM sleep - when you are out like a light and experiencing maximum restorative hormone flow, balancing of brain chemicals, and cellular repair). This cycling of REM into non-REM sleep rotates throughout the night, with each complete cycle believed to last about 90 minutes.

EFFECTS OF SLEEP DEFICIENCY

A recent CDC (Centers for Disease Control and Prevention) study found that an increasing percentage of Americans are seriously deficient in sleep (40 percent of Americans get less than five hours of sleep per night), and an incredible 75 percent of us suffer from some form of sleep difficulty each night. (1, 2)

The way you feel while you're awake depends in part on what happens while you're sleeping. During sleep, your body is working to support healthy brain function and maintain your physical health. Sleep architecture changes with age and is easily susceptible to external and internal disruption. Reduction or disruption of sleep can affect numerous bodily functions varying from body homeostasis to how well you think, react, work, learn, and get along with others. Damage from sleep deficiency can also occur in an instant, such as a car crash, or it can harm you over time. Herewith some of the key effects of sleep deficiency:

- Brain Function: Sleep helps your brain work properly. While you're sleeping, your brain is preparing for the next day. It's forming new pathways to help you learn and remember information. Studies show that a good night's sleep improves learning. Whether you're learning math, how to play the piano, how to perfect your golf swing, or how to drive a car, sleep helps enhance your learning and problem-solving skills. Sleep also helps you pay attention, make decisions, and be creative. Studies also show that sleep deficiency (6 hours or less and even relatively moderate sleep restriction) alters activity in some parts of the brain and can seriously impair waking neurobehavioral functions in healthy adults, including making decisions, concentration, memory, solving problems, controlling emotions and behavior, and coping with change. Sleep deficiency also has been linked to depression, suicide, and risk-taking behavior. (3)

- Weight Gain and Risk of Diabetes: Chronic sleep deficit may lead to weight gain by affecting how your body processes and stores carbohydrates and by altering hormones that affect your appetite and metabolism. Sleep helps maintain a healthy balance of the hormones that make you feel hungry (ghrelin) or full (leptin). When you don't get enough sleep, your level of ghrelin goes up, and your level of leptin goes down. The fluctuation causes you to feel hungrier than when you're well-rested. Sleep also affects how your body reacts to insulin, the hormone that controls your blood glucose (sugar) level. Sleep deficiency results in a higher than normal blood sugar level, which may increase your risk for diabetes. (4, 5)

- Immune Function: Your immune system relies on sleep to stay healthy as well. Your immune system defends your body against foreign or harmful substances. Ongoing sleep deficiency can change the way in which your immune system responds, over-taxing it and preventing it from going through the rejuvenation cycles it needs. You may have noticed in the past, that when you were not getting enough sleep, you may have caught a cold? Adequate sleep helps the immune system function optimally and promotes the release of the hormones that enhance brain and endocrine function.

- Heart Health, Stroke, and Cancer: As above, it appears that not allowing your body to go through the rejuvenation periods it needs has dire effects on other bodily functions as well. Emerging data from several studies suggest that sleep deprivation has major metabolic and cardiovascular consequences and consequently might be a risk factor for poor health in the future. Insufficient sleep can lead to hypertension, elevated stress hormone levels, irregular heartbeat, compromised immune function, and an increased risk for heart disease, stroke, and cancer. (6)

CAUSES OF SLEEP DISRUPTION OR DEPRIVATION

There are several factors that contribute to sleep problems. These factors can be both external and internal. The internal factors affecting our ability to sleep include chronic health issues and chronic mental stress, which can keep you up at night, worrying over problems, deadlines, and frustrations. External factors affecting our sleep include what we eat and drink (sugar, caffeine, too much alcohol), excessive artificial light and digital stimulation after sunset, our sleep environment, the medications that we take, irregular bed and wake times, jet lag, and graveyard shift work. All these factors, individual or combined, can all disrupt sleep patterns. Herewith some of the key causes of sleep disruption:

- Health Issues: A wide range of medical and psychological conditions can have an impact on sleep, including liver disease, heart failure, arthritis, Parkinson's, cancer, and the potential chronic pain from some of them. Other contributors could be discomfort caused by gastroesophageal reflux disease or pre-menstrual syndrome. Being overweight can also contribute to sleep problems such as finding comfortable sleeping positions, sleep apnea, and general body pain. Pain and discomfort tend to limit the depth of sleep and allow only brief episodes of sleep between awakenings.

  People experiencing stress, anxiety, and depression might also make it more difficult to fall asleep, and when they do, sleep tends to be light and includes more REM sleep and less deep sleep. Sleep deprivation is likely because our bodies are programmed to respond to stressful and potentially dangerous situations by waking up. Stress, even that caused by daily concerns, can stimulate this arousal response and make restful sleep more difficult to achieve.

- Medications: Sleep deprivation has also been attributed to the consumption of certain types of medication. These include alpha blockers, beta blockers, anti-depressants, and antihistamines. Drugs can have a hefty impact on what affects sleep patterns. For instance, beta-blockers, which are used to treat conditions such as high blood pressure, glaucoma, heart failure, or migraines, can cause low levels of REM and deep sleep. They are also responsible for causing an increase in daytime sleepiness. The same can be observed with alpha blockers that are used to treat prostate issues and high blood pressure.

- Caffeine: A chemical called adenosine, which builds up in the brain during wakefulness, may be at least partly responsible for sleep drive. As adenosine levels increase, scientists think that the chemical begins to inhibit the brain cells that promote alertness, which gives rise to the sleepiness we experience when we have been awake for many hours. Interestingly, caffeine, the world's most widely used stimulant, works by temporarily blocking the adenosine receptors in these specific parts of the brain. Because these nerve cells cannot sense adenosine in the presence of caffeine, they maintain their activity, and we stay alert. If sleep does occur following the intake of caffeine, the stimulant's effects may persist for some time and can influence the patterns of sleep. For instance, caffeine generally decreases the quantity of slow-wave sleep and REM sleep and tends to increase the number of awakenings. The duration of its effect depends on the amount of caffeine ingested, the amount of time before sleep that the person ingests the caffeine, the individual's tolerance level, the degree of ongoing sleep debt and the phase of the individual's internal clock. Research shows that consuming caffeine up to six hours before bed significantly worsened sleep quality. (7)

- Alcohol: Alcohol is commonly used as a sleep aid. However, although alcohol can help a person fall asleep more quickly, the quality of that individual's sleep under the influence of alcohol will be compromised. Ingesting more than one or two drinks shortly before bedtime has been shown to cause increased awakenings—and in some cases insomnia—due to the arousal effect the alcohol has as it is metabolized later in the night. Alcohol also tends to worsen the symptoms of sleep apnea, which will further disrupt sleep in people with this breathing disorder.

- Sugary Foods: Eating simple carbs is heavily discouraged for all the reasons mentioned in previous chapters, but carbs also affect sleep. They interfere with the body's production of melatonin and cause irregular insulin activity in the body, contributing to sleep arousals – intrusions that pull you out of deep sleep.

Additionally, we are designed to burn fat through the sleep restoration period because it burns long and slow, in contrast to sugar and carbs, which burn quickly. With Western eating habits most people never go into fat metabolism during sleep, instead, because the body is accustomed to it, it attempts to burn sugars during sleep cycles as it did during awake periods. With sugar and short chain carbs delivering only short, quick emergency bursts of energy, sleeping through the night becomes impossible.

- Light: Light can have a significant impact on the sleep cycle. The retinas in our eyes react to light because of the presence of light-sensitive cells. These cells are positioned in the same areas the rods and cones which are responsible for vision. They tell the brain whether it is daytime or nighttime so that it knows when to induce sleep. Unfortunately, since synthetic light sources from indoor lighting such as; computers, TVs, cell phones, iPads, electronic gadgets are all around us, it makes it harder for the brain to process information correctly. The brain can become over-stimulated by all the electronic and digital devices. This can all lead to a confused circadian rhythm, ultimately causing a reduction in our sleep time and or sleep quality.

- The Sleep Environment: The environment in your bedroom can have a significant influence on sleep quality and quantity. Several variables combine to make up the sleep environment, including electronics around your bed and in your room, light, noise, and temperature. Electronics and lights can over-stimulate your brain making it hard to fall asleep and affecting the quality and length of sleep throughout the night. Temperature can also affect the quality and length of sleep. Noises can make it difficult to fall asleep as well as wake you through the night.

- Jet Lag and Night Shift Work: Traveling long distances and through various time zones can cause "jet lag" as our internal clocks have to adjust to changing time zones. The condition can last up to several days, especially if it is day where you have traveled to, and your body clock is on night in your originating time zone. Similarly, with night shift work, you are trying to sleep during the day and work through the night. The body cannot easily adjust to these changes and can go through periods of insomnia when it is time to go to sleep and excessive sleepiness through the periods it needs to be awake.

WAYS TO IMPROVE SLEEP

Good quality sleep is as important as a healthy diet and regular exercise, and as shown earlier in the chapter, poor sleep can have immediate and long-term negative effects on your health. The good news is good sleep is more in your control than you might think. But, to make certain of this, it is critical to create a sleep routine or sleep hygiene (sets of practices, habits, and environmental influences that can improve your ability to fall asleep and stay asleep) and then stick with it. Doctors learn sleep hygiene in medical school or during their residency as they clearly understand they need to have all of their faculties during the long hours they put in during their residencies and following good sleep hygiene can make the difference between success and failure.

Here are some of the key components for creating good sleep hygiene:

- Sleep Environment: Create an area of minimal stimulation and maximum relaxation for sleep. Your bedroom should be used for sleep and sex only, with no computer, television, or work desk present. You should have a clear physical and psychological separation between your bedroom and other areas of the house where you do work or enjoy entertainment. Minimize external noise, light and artificial lights from devices like alarm clocks and make sure your bedroom is a quiet, relaxing, and clean and clear of clutter. Lower the volume of outside noise with earplugs or a "white noise" appliance. Use heavy curtains, blackout shades, or an eye mask to block light. Keep the temperature comfortably cool (between 65 and 70°F) and the room well ventilated. Make sure to have the right mattress, pillows, and bedding to optimize sleep comfort.

- Consistent Sleep Schedule: Establish a consistent, circadian-friendly routine to optimize hormone flows and ensure you enjoy complete sleep cycles. Your body's circadian rhythm functions on a set loop, aligning itself with sunrise and sunset. Remember that melatonin floods your bloodstream on circadian cue triggered by darkness. Going to bed and waking up at the same time each day sets the body's "internal clock" to expect sleep at a certain time night after night. Try to stick as closely as possible to your routine on weekends to avoid a Monday morning sleep hangover.

- Pre-Sleep Routine: It is important to wind down calmly in the hours preceding your bedtime. Minimize your central nervous system stimulation before going to bed, so you can have a smooth, relaxing transition from your busy day to downtime. Ease the transition from wake time to sleep time with a period of relaxing activities an hour or so before bed. Light reading, listening to relaxing music, taking a hot bath, deep breathing and visualization, and relaxation techniques before bed can all help relax you and improve sleep quality.

- Reduce Caffeine: Try not to drink more than two caffeinated drinks (coffee or caffeinated tea) per day and ensure you only drink them in the morning or up until mid-day. When consumed late in the day, the stimulation of your nervous system may stop your body from naturally relaxing at night. Caffeine can stay elevated in the blood for 6–8 hours so drinking coffee or tea late in the day is not recommended. If you do crave a cup of coffee or tea in the late afternoon or evening, then stick with decaffeinated coffee or herbal tea.

- Day Light Exposure: As highlighted earlier in the chapter, your body has a natural time-keeping clock known as your circadian rhythm. It affects your brain, body, and hormones, helping you stay awake and telling your body when it's time to sleep. Natural sunlight or bright light during the day helps keep your circadian rhythm healthy, and it also helps improve daytime energy, as well as nighttime sleep quality and duration. Get at least two hours of bright light exposure every day.

- Reduce Blue Light at Night: Exposure to light during the day is beneficial, but nighttime light exposure has the opposite effect. Again, this is due to its impact on your circadian rhythm, tricking your brain into thinking it is still daytime. The effect reduces hormones like melatonin, which helps you relax and get deep sleep, and blue light is the worst in this regard, which emits in large amounts from electronic devices like smartphones and computers. Try to avoid using these devices at night, which I understand is impractical for many of us. If that is the case and you absolutely have to use them at night download an app such as f.lux (https://justgetflux.com) to block the blue light on your computer. I use f.lux as I often have to work at night and I can tell you it definitely helps. There are similar blue light blocker apps for iPhones and Android phones. Examine your 'app stores' for them. Lastly, blue light blocking glasses are available, which I have not tried personally, but understand they are effective.

- Irregular and Long Naps: Short "power naps" can be beneficial, but long or irregular napping during the day can negatively affect your sleep as sleeping in the daytime can confuse your internal body clock. If you are accustomed to taking regular daytime naps and your sleep is not affected at night than don't change a thing.

- Eating: Do not eat late as that can negatively impact both sleep quality and the natural release of growth hormone and melatonin. Stick with the eating plan in the program and you will be fine.

- Exercise: Regular exercise has many health benefits as discussed in the *Exercise* chapter. The benefits also include improving sleep. It is best to workout earlier in the day or up until the early evening as performing it too late in the day may cause problems falling asleep for some people due to the stimulatory effect of it, as it increases alertness and hormones like epinephrine or adrenaline.

Optional:

- Alcohol: If you enjoy wine try to stick with having one glass with dinner, which also may help you relax and unwind in the evening hours. The earlier the better to provide your body time to metabolize the alcohol before bedtime. Do not drink just before bed as that can increase awakenings as mentioned in the 'causes of sleep disruptions' section of this chapter.

- Diffuser: Using a diffuser in your room with a few drops of organic lavender essential oil can also help you sleep better. If you try this make sure to get a diffuser that has no lights and one that is quiet. Some of them also make hissing sounds some people find relaxing.

- Melatonin: A melatonin supplement is an extremely popular aid to fall asleep faster and improve sleep quality. If you want to try it start with a 2mg dosage and see how you respond to it. I travel quite a lot internationally and always take melatonin on my trips as I find that it helps me acclimate faster to the new time zones. I personally use the Natrol brand.

- Chamomile Tea: Chamomile tea is touted for its mild sedative effect, and many people feel it helps them relax and ease into sleep better.

Closing Note

The amount of sleep recommended by the US Department of Health and Human Services and the National Sleep Foundation for optimal health and biological function for adults is 7-9 hours.

10

Your Best Skin

"The secret of change is to focus all of your energy, not on fighting the old, but on building the new."

~ SOCRATES

Every element of this program is designed to work synergistically and contribute to age reversal, but if I had to place one thing as the single most important component for your skin, it would be what we introduce through our mouths to our bodies. Considering the skin is the largest organ, shouldn't it receive the amount of attention it deserves?

The total skin surface of an adult ranges from 12 to 20 square feet and comprises about 15% of the body's weight. Its chemical composition is about 70% water, 25% protein, 2% lipids with the remainder made up of trace minerals, nucleic acids, glycosaminoglycans, proteoglycans, and numerous other chemicals.

The skin consists of three main layers. The visible layer is the epidermis which is made up of four different kinds of skin cells; keratinocytes, melanocytes, Merkel cells, and Langerhans cells. The dermis composed of proteins (like collagen and elastin) supports the skin. The hypodermis often called subcutaneous tissue is primarily made of fat for insulation and support for the skin's the upper layers.

Protection is a major function of the skin, and it is the body's primary physical barrier against infection and disease. But, there are other functions of this vital organ as well. The skin is full of nerve endings that help sense things around you. It emits sweat when you're hot; sweat evaporating from the skin cools the body. The skin acts like a sack holding much of the body's critical fluids and nutrients. Biologically, the skin is the first line of defense; culturally, skin defines much of our standard of beauty. Radiant, youthful skin signals healthy and vitality.

INTERNAL DAMAGE

As highlighted in other chapters of the book, lifestyle choices are not only causing us to age prematurely, but causing us to get sick and diseased, and those toxic factors deliver devastating effects to our skin. What we put into our mouths and bodies can cause inflammation throughout the body, and this triggers many other biological responses including inflammation, oxidative stress, mitochondria malfunction, and glycation. These are all related reactions that compromise the body's natural state of balance. They manifest themselves as aging throughout the body's organ systems and are most apparent in the skin.

Mitochondria Malfunction

Mitochondria are the fuel factories in our cells that create cellular energy (ATP). When mitochondria malfunction, cells die. How well we age, including our vulnerability to disease is due in part to how healthy our mitochondria are. Recent studies have linked oxidative stress (the accumulation of free radicals in the cell) and genetic defects in mitochondria with premature aging. In this case, I am talking about chronological aging, it's cellular, or biological aging means that the DNA inside a healthy cell has become fragmented or shortened, which affects the mitochondria inside the cell. (1, 2)

Glycation

The wrong kinds of carbs and omega 6s in our diets contribute hugely to dysfunctional biological processes. Besides inflammation, too much sugar and other "junk" like processed, simple carb foods, ultimately lead to a metabolic process called glycation (or glycosylation). Glycation is the process in which sugar molecules in the blood ultimately bond to proteins and DNA and over time become chemically modified.

The new bonded proteins are called "advanced glycation end-products," ironically identified as AGEs for short. AGEs create unnatural crosslinks with collagen and elastin proteins that support the dermis, altering their shape, flexibility, elasticity, and function rendering them incapable of easy repair. What's more, the presence of AGE's generates additional inflammation.

Glycation is one of the major molecular mechanisms whereby damage accrues throughout your body and leads to disease and aging. This process is accelerated in all body tissues when sugar is elevated. The damage is further stimulated by ultraviolet light in the skin. (3)

Oxidative Stress

Oxidative stress occurs when the body does not have enough antioxidants to neutralize free radicals. Free Radicals are atoms, ions, or molecules that contain an unpaired electron. The unpaired electron makes them unstable and highly reactive. In a process called oxidation, free radicals steal electrons from other molecules in fats, proteins, cell membranes, and even DNA, altering the fundamental structure of the affected molecule. One unbalanced molecule may not sound like a major concern, but oxidation sets off a chain reaction by damaging a cell's DNA, structure, and ability to function. Over time, oxidative damage accumulates and contributes to aging and a variety of degenerative diseases.

What's causing the overabundance of free radicals? The answer is easy to guess. A major contributor is poor lifestyle choices, which includes diet (junk foods, processed, GMO foods, simple carbs, sugars, omega 6s, chemical additives, etc.), smoking*, prescription medications, and heavily chemically treated drinking water. Environmental factors play a role as well. (4, 5)

*If you are a smoker, I urge you to stop immediately. We all know that smoking is bad and it causes so many life-threatening diseases; cancer, emphysema, heart disease -- the list of dangers is long. Smoking also happens to be the second leading cause of premature aging, following sun damage. Every time you inhale cigarette smoke billions of free radicals invade your body ultimately breaking down the collagen and elastin in your skin. This effect results in sagging, wrinkled skin that continues to worsen over time. Within a few months of smoking cessation and full incorporation of my program, you may drop as much as ten years off of your appearance. I hope that is incentive enough to quit!

EXTERNAL DAMAGE

UV Light

We often associate a tanned, glowing complexion with good health. That perception is far from the truth. Skin color obtained from being in the sun, or from a tanning booth, actually accelerates the skin's aging and increases the risk of developing skin cancer.

The skin uses sunlight to help manufacture vitamin D, which is critical for overall health. Vitamin D is also beneficial in controlling some chronic skin diseases such as psoriasis. It promotes a sense of well-being, but ultraviolet (UV) light from sunlight and tanning beds can also cause significant damage to the skin.

UV light, although invisible to the human eye, is a component of sunlight, or light from tanning beds. UV light also has the most adverse effect on the skin. There are three classifications of UV light; UVA, UVB, and UVC -- all three cause damage. UV radiation is one of the creators of free radicals. Free radicals cause a chain reaction that damage cells on a molecular level, including DNA. They not only increase the number of enzymes that break down collagen, but they can also alter a cell's genetic material in a way that can lead to cancer.

Sun exposure causes most of the skin changes that we think of as a normal part of aging. Over time, the sun's UV light also damages the fibers in the skin called elastin. When these fibers deteriorate, the skin begins to sag, stretch, and lose its ability to go back into place after stretching. The skin also bruises and tears more easily, taking longer to heal. So while sun damage to the skin may not be apparent when you're young, it will appear later in life.

Some of the skin related damages caused by over-exposure to UV include:

- Pre-cancerous skin lesions: Actinic keratosis.
- Cancerous skin lesions: Basal cell carcinoma, squamous cell carcinoma, and melanoma.
- Benign tumors.
- Fine and coarse wrinkles.
- Freckles.
- Discolored areas of the skin: mottled pigmentation.
- Sallowness: A yellow discoloration of the skin.

- Telangiectasia (spider veins): Small dilated blood vessels near the surface of the skin.
- Elastosis: The destruction of the elastic and collagen tissue (causing lines, wrinkles, and sagging skin).

Other Environmental Aggressors

Most people are exposed to environmental stressors every day. Common elements like; infrared radiation from electromagnetic radiation – radio waves, ultraviolet radiation, X-rays, and microwaves are invisible to the human eye. Pollution also contributes to the subsistence of free radicals. These aggressors lead to the same place as the other contributors mentioned earlier; inflammation, damaged DNA, and oxidative stress.

Personal Care Products

The cosmetic industry is loosely regulated in the US and there are many chemicals allowed in personal care products that research has proven to be harmful. Groups such as the Environment Working Group - Skin Deep Cosmetics Database (EWG) and the National Institutes of Environmental Health Science (NIEHS) do vital research on the safety of the chemicals we are exposed to in our daily lives. Their research is now proving that harsh chemicals like parabens, sulfates phthalates, propylene and polyethylene glycols, BHA, BHT, EDTA, mineral oils, synthetic fragrances and dyes, as well as many others chemicals that are so commonly used in today's most popular personal care products, can have adverse effects on our health, including allergic reactions such as skin irritations, asthma, organ and cellular toxicity, disruption of the endocrine function, which can cause hormone disruption, potentially impair fertility, and even contribute to breast cancer.

Further to the above, many of these chemicals breed free radicals, causing further damage to our skin and negating any product claim of being "youth-enhancing."

The prevalence of petroleum-based chemicals in toiletries and cosmetics is even more troubling. One ubiquitous category called "phthalates" is shown to have several potential health risks associated with exposure.

In the next segment, I provide examples of 'clean' and safe ingredients and products to maximize skin health from the inside-out and the outside-in.

RESTORATION AND PREVENTION

Earlier in this book I highlighted the impact our lifestyles have on skin and how we look extrinsically. In this section I focus on the synergistic things that unveil your absolute best skin -- the skin nature intended for you.

Inside – Out

What you eat and drink has a tremendous impact on your skin. Terrific skin definitely starts from the inside. Providing the right nutrients optimizes the body's ability to perform its natural biological functions, which in turn promotes healthier cells throughout the body, ultimately manifesting itself extrinsically with healthier, younger looking skin.

Diet

Follow the plan from the *Nutritional Intake* chapter, which highlights plenty of superfoods like rich, deep-colored vegetables and fruits, as well as quality fats and proteins. Nutrient rich-brightly colored organic foods are vital for their anti-oxidant benefits and are especially crucial to counteract free radicals. The immune system relies on antioxidants to defend cells from free radicals. Anti-oxidants neutralize free radicals and quench minor inflammation by sacrificing one of their electrons without adverse effect. Since free radicals are inescapable, our bodies should have a constant supply of antioxidant nutrients to keep skin cells healthy, and whole foods are the best place to get them.

The *Supplements* chapter covers exceptions for the use of supplements like astaxanthin. As clearly mentioned there, I do not recommend supplemental forms of antioxidants. I prefer getting them from whole foods, which the body can effectively assimilate, recognizing the molecular structure as nature intended, unlike synthesized, manufactured supplements.

The right types of fats are also imperative as they build and retain moisture in the skin from the inside-out. They boost biological processes such as cell renewal and even help plump skin layers. Essential fatty acids from 'good fats' also have an anti-inflammatory effect on the body, especially Omega-3 derived from wild caught sockeye salmon.

Good proteins have skin benefits as well, including boosting fibroblast production such as collagen and elastin, assisting with cell renewal, and keeping important muscle below the skin surface fit and healthy. Protein's contribution helps with skin tautness as well.

Eating probiotic rich foods will boost beneficial anti-inflammatory flora in the digestive tract, which also helps with the assimilation of nutrients and allows for optimal cell health.

Water

Is quite literally, the river on which our good health flows. Without enough water, your skin loses elasticity, becomes dry, and your body doesn't function optimally. Water carries nutrients to our cells, aids digestion by forming stomach secretions, flushes the body of wastes, and keeps the kidneys healthy. Water keeps our moisture-rich organs (skin, eyes, mouth, and nose) functioning well. It lubricates and cushions joints, regulates body temperatures, metabolism, and boosts blood circulation. It promotes efficient use of all the body's systems and delivers a healthier, more radiant appearance to the skin.

Dehydration is a big problem if you are trying to promote your best skin. Make sure to drink enough water every day. Try to consume 8-10 glasses of purified water a day.

Supplements: There are a few supplements that will benefit the skin - follow my recommendations in the *Supplements* chapter. Astaxanthin, the right vitamin D, omega-3, and collagen all have wonderful skin benefits.

Avoids: As recommended in the *Nutritional Intake* plan, stay away from ingredients that promote inflammation such as sugar and simple carbohydrates, soft drinks, artificial sweeteners, omega-6 fats, and food additives. Limit caffeine intake as well as that can act as a diuretic and dehydrate you.

Intermittent Fasting (IF)

Will give your system a rest and help cleanse and detox, which boosts overall cell health, including those in the skin.

Outside – In

What we put inside our bodies ranks highest on the intervention scale, but care from the outside is still necessary and plays an important role too. I like to think of the holistic benefits of feeding my skin from the inside-out and the outside-in.

Earlier in this chapter, I highlighted the plethora of harsh chemicals hidden in skin care products and the potential risks they pose. The risks are real, and ideally, such chemicals should be eliminated from use. It is important to note that there are many clinically proven ingredients that have fantastic efficacies that are safe.

As mentioned in the *Introduction*, one of the founding philosophies at *Nutrimax* was to ensure all of the raw materials used for our products were 'food state,' meaning the molecular structure was similar to the values of nutrients found in whole foods and with similar bioavailability. This allowed the body to fully absorb and utilize the nutrients with ease and without any damage to the body by way of toxic buildup or free radical and inflammation causation. I enacted the same philosophy entering the skin care industry in 2001. While we were committed to efficacy and results, every ingredient chosen had to be compatible with the body's natural biological processes. We strived to ensure every additive was 'clean' and had no adverse effects, whatsoever.

The 'purity rule' still tops the list of our brand philosophies today. We only manufacture effective and safe skin care products that are clean and free of harsh chemicals and are committed to health and safety with a standard that goes above and beyond what is legally required in the US.

Here are a few good examples of how you can create wonders for your skin inexpensively:

Moisturize

You can make rich moisturizers at home using organic cold-pressed coconut, rosehip seed, avocado, or argon oils and hyaluronic acid (HA). These oils are rich in nutrients such as essential fatty acids (EFAs), vitamins and anti-oxidants. They are highly absorbable, have rich moisturizing properties, and many anti-aging skin benefits. HA provides a moisture-binding characteristic that helps the skin retain water. One of the qualities of youthful skin is its ability to hold water and distribute the balanced amount of moisture. As we age, our skin loses that ability, resulting in a visible loss of firmness, pliability, and diminished appearance of plumpness and suppleness. HA helps to plump the skin, smoothing fines lines and wrinkles.

Depending on your skin type and desired level of richness by increasing or decreasing the drops of oil (example: for a day moisturizer, add a drop or two of your preferred oil and several drops of HA). Rub your hands together to blend and heat and massage oil fully into cleansed skin. For a night moisturizer, try a little heavier application of oil or mix a blend of oils using one or two drops of each. Add the HA or use the oil on its own depending on your personal preference. I recommend moisturizing morning and night, every day.

I like the idea of blending the HA with the oils both morning and night as it creates a serum of sorts. If you use organic, cold-pressed coconut oil, the likelihood of it being solid VS liquid is quite high. It can be smoothed into the skin this way, but it may prove easier to put a little dab in the palm of your hand, then rub both hands together, which will immediately liquefy the solid oil. Lastly, always cleanse skin before application of any topical product. Use a gentle, clean cleanser, free of harsh chemicals. If you choose to buy a HA serum avoid any that also contain alcohol, parabens, sulfates, or other ingredients that are harmful to the skin. Try to find a natural one with a clean base.

Protect

As explained earlier in the chapter, the leading cause of premature aging is sun exposure. To prevent skin cancer, premature wrinkling, age spots, and other adverse effects from UV rays wear a 'clean' SPF sunscreen of at least 30 that has both UVA and UVB protection.

Applying sunscreen is my least favorite skin care protocol. Most commercial sunscreen lotions feel thick, heavy, and clogging on the skin. I prefer to use natural, micronized zinc-based products and stay clear of the heavy chemical-based, highly commercial brands. Mineral based powders may also provide an alternative option for protection, personally have only tried the powder a few times.

Exfoliate

The skin is a passageway that rids our body of toxins and helps prevent chemical and waste build-up. Clear pores enable your body to expel waste such as toxins that accumulate in our bodies. Pores that are congested and blocked with chemicals and pollutants prevent skin from functioning properly and removing toxins.

Pores can also become blocked with dead skin cells, preventing normal sebum excretion. Blocked pores cause a buildup of sebum under the skin and lead to whiteheads, blackheads, and pimples. Failure to exfoliate gives the skin a grayish tone and overall look of dullness.

Exfoliating regularly will keep pores clean and clear as well as encourage cell renewal giving way to a more youthful looking skin. I do not like the popular, physical exfoliators like face scrubs or heavy chemical versions of alpha hydroxy acids (AHA) and beta hydroxy acids (BHA). I believe many of these products are too harsh on the delicate skin. They strip away dead skin cells, but in doing so, they also remove newer cells. AHAs and BHA that are too strong may cause skin irritation.

What is the difference between AHA and BHA? Alpha hydroxy acids are water soluble, while beta hydroxy acids are lipid (oil) soluble. Beta hydroxy acid can penetrate the sebum pores, and exfoliate the dead skin cells that are built up inside the pore. Beta hydroxy acid is preferable for oily skin because of its difference in properties. As for enzymes, they work similarly to both AHA and BHA, but they are typically gentler on the skin. Enzymes have a proteolytic effect (the breakdown of proteins into smaller polypeptides or amino acids) and induce superficial exfoliation of the stratum corneum cells.

I recommend natural fruit/food derived AHAs, BHAs, and enzymes for exfoliation. Make a paste or puree using a variety of fresh ingredients; lemons, grapefruit, mango, cucumber, and tomatoes all of which contain AHA's; strawberries and raspberries contain AHA and salicylic acid, which is a BHA. Papaya and pineapple are rich in natural enzymes, bromelain, papain, and they contain AHAs. Yogurt delivers lactic acid -- a natural AHA and apples contain malic acid, also a natural AHA. Blend any of these ingredients together for a fantastic, safe and efficacious home treatment. Use once or twice a week and leave on the skin for approximate 20 mins each treatment.

I understand there is some work that goes into the do-it-yourself approach to skin-care products. It is certainly more convenient to buy something off the shelf. If you decide to buy commercially available products, read the labels. Try to select compounds containing ingredients with plant derived AHA/BHA or enzymes and do not contain the harsh chemicals we have mentioned. I use a Skin Moderne product from the Elemental line called AHA/BHA. The base of AHA/BHA is a clean foundation of hyaluronic acid and the product contains no harsh chemicals, so it is mild on the skin.

Treatments

Anti-aging serums containing ingredients like peptides and growth factors can certainly be useful. Much of the results depends on the level of actives and what other ingredients are in the product, including the harsh chemicals mentioned throughout this chapter. There is plenty of solid clinical evidence validating the efficacies of epidermal growth factors (EFG) and various types of peptides. If used at the appropriate clinical levels and in clean bases, I would strongly recommend them for adults 35 or older. The problem is finding a commercially prepared product containing the actives at clinical levels and in clean bases. If you know you are getting these two areas covered, then, by all means, go for it. I use a serum with these actives daily.

Additional Factors

Exercise

I highlighted so many benefits in the *Exercise = Life Extension* chapter, but intentionally left one out so I can include it here. As it turns out, physical activity not only appears to keep skin younger, it may also even reverse skin aging in people who start exercising late in life.

Skin changes as we get older; wrinkles and crow's feet form, uneven pigmentation appears, the skin's tone dulls, and sagging areas are more apparent. Most visible issues are the result of changes within the layers of skin. At about age 40, most of us begin to experience a thickening of the stratum corneum - the outer layer of the epidermis (the top layer of your skin). The stratum corneum is the portion of the skin you see and feel. It is composed mostly of dead skin cells and some collagen, so it gets naturally drier, flakier, and dense with age.

About the same time in the biological process, the layer of skin beneath the epidermis, the dermis, begins to thin. It loses cells and elasticity creating a translucent and sagging appearance.

Mark Tarnopolsky, MD, Ph.D. and a team of researchers from McMaster University in Hamilton, Canada, conducted two independent studies to ascertain the effects of exercise on the skin. The *New York Times* featured an article in 2014 on the team's remarkable published results.

The first research trial involved 29 male and female volunteers ages 20 to 84. About half of the participants were active, performing at least three hours of moderate to vigorous physical activity every week. The remaining half of the volunteer study participants were resolutely sedentary, exercising for less than an hour per week.

Comparing before and after biopsies taken from the buttock area, researchers found that after age 40, the men and women who exercised frequently had markedly thinner, healthier stratum corneum and thicker dermis layers in their skin. Their skin was much closer in composition to that of the 20-and 30-year-olds study participants than to that of others within their age group, even if they were past age 65.

The researchers considered other factors that may have played a role in the results, including diet, genes, and lifestyles between the exercising and sedentary groups. They felt it was impossible to know for sure if exercise exclusively affected people's skin or the results were incidental to lucky genetics and healthier lives. So the researchers studied a group of sedentary volunteers. They first obtained skin samples from their buttocks, then prescribed an exercise program.

The volunteers in the follow-up, aged 65 or older, at the study's start. They all had "normal skin" for their age. The study participants began a structured endurance training program, working out twice a week, jogging or cycling at a moderately strenuous pace, equivalent to at least 65 percent of their maximum aerobic capacity for 30 minutes. The exercise program continued for three months. At the end of that trial, the researchers again biopsied the volunteers' skin.

The second biopsy samples looked quite different from the initial, pre-study biopsies. The outer and inner layers of the study group's skin looked very similar to those of 20- to 40-year-olds. "I don't want to over-hype the results but it was pretty remarkable to see," said Dr. Tarnopolsky. Under a microscope, the volunteers' skin "looked like that of a much younger person, and all that they had done differently was exercise."

The researches were unclear about the exact biological processes that contributed to these fantastic results, but some of the things that stuck out include; better mitochondrial function, higher levels of a free radical scavenger within the mitochondria called superoxide dismutase 2 (an antioxidant the body naturally produces), and higher levels of a cytokine called interleukin-15 (IL-15). The volunteers' skin samples contained almost 50 percent more IL-15 after they had been exercising than at the start of the study. (6, 7, 8)

Stress

Your emotions have a powerful effect on your skin. They can cause skin issues to flare up regardless of what you're prone to, whether it's acne, psoriasis, or eczema. Stress releases cortisol, which can throw off the other hormones in your body and cause the skin to look tired, gray, blotchy, and even cause you to breakout.

Stress is a natural occurrence in life. It happens to everyone. Since you can't avoid your job, bills, or other life experiences, the best thing to do is learn to manage stress. It is possible to minimize the effects by eating healthy, exercising regularly, getting enough sleep, and taking care of yourself in general. Yoga, breathing exercises, and meditation can also help manage stress.

Sleep

Sleep plays a tremendous role in how good – or bad our skin looks. Proper sleep ensures optimal biological processes, including cell renewal. The body when deprived of sleep it goes into a state of stress, producing cortisol, and as indicated, this can cause the skin to look tired, gray, blotchy, and cause breakouts.

11

Connection = Happiness & Longevity?
(Bonus Chapter)

"No man is an island."

~ **John Dunne**

The subject of happiness and how it contributes to longevity was not part of my initial thinking nor was it included in the original outline for this book. While writing, I read an intriguing article and then watched a Ted Talk feature about *The Harvard Study of Adult Development* (also called *The Harvard Grant Study* or *The Harvard Grant & Glueck Study*). My interest piqued, so I explored the subject further. There is such compelling research connecting happiness and longevity that I felt compelled to add a chapter highlighting the contribution.

The Harvard Study of Adult Development tracked the physical and emotional well-being of 268 male graduates from Harvard University, as well as 456 poor men growing up in Boston from 1939 to 2014. Most of the Harvard subjects entered the study from more or less the same point of emotional maturity in life. One segment of the study consisted of successful, happy, men who led a full, rewarding life (not necessarily at the same time). The other segment consisted of men whose life experiences included failures, misery, and loneliness, and painful deaths. In 2015 the study continued under the name of a second-generation study and the research was expanded to include the wives and children of the original study group.

The unique study measured and recorded nearly every life experience including; physical and psychological fitness, family background, career development, marriages, and divorces. Multiple generations of researchers analyzed brain scans, blood samples, self-reported surveys, and interactions with these men to compile their findings.

Current surveys show that most young adults believe obtaining wealth and fame are the keys to a happy and healthy life. The Harvard study suggests the essential forecast of aging well and experiencing a long and happy life is not the amount of money you amass or the notoriety you receive. The best and most important barometer of long-term health and well-being is the strength of relationships with family, friends, and spouses.

The Harvard Study revealed close relationships, not money or fame, served to keep people happy throughout their lives. Positive personal relationships protect people from life's discontents, help to delay mental and physical decline, and are better predictors of long and happy lives than social class, IQ, or even genes. The findings proved true across the board among both the Harvard men and the inner-city participants. The on-going study spanning almost 80 years indicates embracing a close community helps people live longer, happier lives.

Robert Waldinger, a Harvard clinical professor of psychiatry and the fourth director of *The Harvard Study of Adult Development* summarizes:

The conclusions are simple, close relationships can make or break a person's well-being. Good relationships keep us happier and healthier. Period. If you want to be happier and healthier in the coming year, invest in close, positive relationships. Having someone to lean on keeps brain function high and reduces emotional and even physical pain. People who feel lonely are more likely to experience health declines earlier in life, and they tend to die sooner.

> The surprising finding is that our relationships and how happy we are in our relationships have a powerful influence on our health. Taking care of your body is important, but tending to your relationships is a form of self-care too. That, I think, is the revelation. Good relationships don't just protect our bodies; they protect our brains, and those good relationships, they don't have to be smooth all the time. Some of our octogenarian couples could bicker with each other day in and day out, but as long as they felt that they could really count on the other when the going got tough, those arguments didn't take a toll on their memories. The good life is built on good relationships.

The Harvard study also showed that the role of genetics and long-lived ancestors proved less important to longevity than the level of satisfaction with relationships in midlife, now recognized as an accurate predictor of healthy aging. "Genes are good, but joy is better," observed one of the study's researchers. The research also debunked the idea that people's personalities are "set like plaster" by age 30 and cannot be changed.

George Vaillant, a Harvard psychiatrist and third director of the study from 1972 to 2004 writes:

> Those [men] who were clearly train wrecks when they were in their 20s turned out to be wonderful octogenarians. On the other hand, alcoholism and major depression could take people who started life as stars and leave them at the end of their lives as train wrecks.

Vaillant wrote a book about the study's findings titled *Triumphs of Experience: The Men of the Harvard Grant Study*. In an article published by *The Huffington Post* (The 75-Year Study that Found the Secrets to a

Fulfilling Life," August 23, 2013) writer Carolyn Gregoire synthesized five key elements from Vaillant's work:

Love is REALLY All That Matters

Gregoire's article points out, "It may seem obvious, but that doesn't make it any less true - love is key to a happy and fulfilling life." She stresses Vaillant's writing, "There are two pillars of happiness; one is love, the other is finding a way of coping with life that does not push love away. The study's most significant finding is that the only thing that matters in life is relationships. A man could have a successful career, money and good physical health, but without supportive, loving relationships, he wouldn't be happy. Happiness is only the cart; love is the horse."

It's About More than Money and Power

The Grant Study's findings echoed those of other studies that acquiring more money and power doesn't correlate to greater happiness. That's not to say money or traditional career success don't matter. But they're small parts of a much larger picture, and while they may loom large for us at the moment, they diminish in importance when viewed in the context of a full life. Gregoire quotes Vaillant's words:

> We found that contentment in the late 70s was not even suggestively associated with the parental social class or even the man's own income. In terms of achievement, the only thing that matters is that you be content at your work.

Regardless of How We Begin Life, We Can All Become Happier

Vaillant describes the case of a man named Godfrey Minot Camille:

> Camille went into the Grant study with fairly bleak prospects for life satisfaction. Camille had the lowest rating for the future

stability of all the subjects, and he had previously attempted suicide. But at the end of his life, he was one of the happiest. Why? As Vaillant explains, He spent his life searching for love.

Connection Is Crucial

According to Vaillant, "Joy is the connection. The more areas in your life you can make a connection, the better." The study found strong relationships to be far and away the strongest predictor of life satisfaction. Regarding career satisfaction, feeling connected to one's work was far more important than making money or achieving traditional success. The conclusion of the study, not in a medical but in a psychological sense, is that "connection is the whole shooting match," says Vaillant. It is evident as life goes on, relationship connections become even more important. The Grant Study provides strong support for the growing body of research that links social ties with longevity, lowers stress levels, and improves overall well-being.

Challenges and the Perspective They Give You Can Make You Happier

Vaillant writes:

> The journey from immaturity to maturity is a sort of movement from narcissism to connection, and a big part of this shift has to do with the way we deal with challenges. Coping mechanisms – 'the capacity to make gold out of shit' -- have a significant effect on social support and overall well-being. The secret is replacing narcissism, a single-minded focus on one's own emotional oscillations and perceived problems, with mature coping defenses.

Vaillant concedes, "There are some additional notable findings from the Harvard study. Some factors might seem obvious today, but some attributes are overlooked:

Childhood relationships matter a lot. Men who had 'warm' childhood relationships with their mothers earned $87,000 more money a year, were more effective at work, and were less likely to develop dementia than men who didn't. Men who had 'warm' childhood relationships with their fathers were also more likely to show lower rates of adult anxiety, greater enjoyment of vacations, and increased 'life satisfaction' at age 75. Valliant sums up this point in four words: *"Happiness is love. Period."* (1, 2, 3)

So, what are some of the personal applications of this study if we want to lead long, happy lives? Build and keep warm and healthy relations with friends and family; understand that money doesn't necessarily make a person happy; if you drink, drink moderately, if you smoke, quit; and last but certainly not least -- plan to transform and progress constantly until you die.

Closing note

Interestingly, relationships in Paleolithic times were critical for survival. Without an extended support circle, life expectancy was even shorter. Friends in Paleolithic times depended on one another, and they lived in close-knit communities. Friends were people with whom they went hunting for food. Groups survived long journeys and brutal winters together. They took care of one another when one member fell sick, and they shared their last morsels of food together in times of need. Although it was a different era, connection with other humans was essential for survival. Studying the ancient history of humans and taking into account the Harvard research on adult development, there is convincing evidence that connections are indeed a basic human need. Without a connection to others, happiness, and by extension, longevity, is not achievable. From my perspective, healthy relationship connections certainly appear to generate happiness and longevity!

INTRODUCTION: SOWING THE SEEDS
BOOKS OF INFLUENCE:

1) Bailey, Covert. *Fit or Fat?* Sphere, 1985.
2) Pearson, Durk and Shaw, Sandy. *Life Extension: a Practical Scientific Approach.* Warner Books, 1983.
3) Haas, Robert. *Eat to Win: the Sports, Nutrition, Bible.* Rawson Associates, 1983.
4) Diamond, Harvey, and Marilyn Diamond. *Fit for Life.* Wellness Central, 2010.
5) Kowalski, Robert E. *The 8-Week Cholesterol Cure: How to Lower Your Blood Cholesterol by up to 40 Percent without Drugs or Deprivation.* HarperLargePrint, 2000.
6) Chopra, Deepak. *Ageless Body, Timeless Mind: the Quantum Alternative to Growing Old.* Three Rivers Press, 2010.
7) D'Adamo, Peter. *Eat Right 4 Your Type: the Individualized Blood Type Diet Solution.* New American Library, 2016.
8) Phillips, Bill, and Michael D'Orso. *Body for Life: 12 Weeks to Mental and Physical Strength.* Thorsons, 2002.
9) Price, Weston A. *Nutrition and Physical Degeneration: a Comparison of Primitive and Modern Diets and Their Effects.* Benediction Classics, 2010.

10) Garcia, Oz, and Sharyn Kolberg. *Look and Feel Fabulous Forever: the World's Best Supplements, Anti-Aging Techniques, and High-Tech Health Secrets.* Regan Books, 2002.

11) Berger, Stuart. *Dr. Berger's Immune Power Diet.* Schwartz, 1989.

12) Campbell, T. Colin. *The China Study: the Most Comprehensive Study of Nutrition Ever Conducted and the Startling Implications for Diet, Weight Loss and Long-Term Health.* BenBella Books, Inc., 2016.

13) Small, Gary W., and Gigi Vorgan. *The Longevity Bible: 8 Essential Strategies for Keeping Your Mind Sharp and Your Body Young.* Hyperion Books, 2007.

14) Weil, Andrew. *Healthy Aging: a Lifelong Guide to Your Physical and Spiritual Well-Being.* Anchor, 2007.

15) Friedan, Betty. *Fountain of Age.* Simon & Schuster, 2006.

16) Giampapa, Vincent C., et al. *The Gene Makeover: the 21st Century Anti-Aging Breakthrough.* Basic Health Publications, 2007.

17) Butler, Robert N. *The Longevity Revolution: the Benefits and Challenges of Living a Long Life.* PublicAffairs, 2010.

18) Abrahams, Ruby. *At the End of the Day: Positive & Creative Aging After Midlife.* Eloquent Books, 2008.

19) Hanson, Amy. *Baby Boomers and beyond: Tapping the Ministry Talents and Passions of Adults over Fifty.* Jossey-Bass, 2010.

20) Green, Brent. *Generation Reinvention: How Boomers Today Are Changing Business, Marketing, Aging and the Future.* IUniverse, 2010.

21) Perricone, Nicholas. *The Wrinkle Cure: Unlock the Power of Cosmeceuticals for Supple, Youthful Skin.* Warner Books/Rodale, 2005.

22) Perricone, Nicholas, and Robb Webb. *The Perricone Prescription: a Physician's 28-Day Program for Total Body and Face Rejuvenation.* Harperaudio, 2008.

23) Perricone, Nicholas. *The Perricone Promise: Look Younger, Live Longer in Three Easy Steps.* Time Warner, 2006.

24) Perricone, Nicholas. *Forever Young The Science of Nutrigenomics for Glowing, Wrinkle-Free Skin and Radiant Health at Every Age.* Pocket Books, 2010.

25) Sisson, Mark. *The Primal Blueprint: 21-Day Total Body Transformation.* Primal Blueprint Publishing, 2009.

26) Buettner, Dan. *The Blue Zones: Lessons for Living Longer from the People Who've Lived the Longest.* National Geographic Society, 2009.

27) Perlmutter, David. *Grain Brain: the Surprising Truth about Wheat, Carbs, and Sugar--Your Brain's Silent Killers.* Little Brown, 2015.

28) Perlmutter, David, and Kristin Loberg. *Brain Maker: the Power of Gut Microbes to Heal and Protect Your Brain - for Life.* Yellow Kite, 2015.

29) Gifford, Bill. *Spring Chicken: Stay Young Forever (or Die Trying).* Grand Central Publishing, 2016.

CHAPTER 1: A DOCTOR'S DISCOVERY

1) "Home." *The Weston A. Price Foundation*, The Weston A. Price Foundation, www.westonaprice.org/.

CHAPTER 2: IMPACT OF OUR LIFESTYLES

1) Suez, Jotham, et al. "Artificial Sweeteners Induce Glucose Intolerance by Altering the Gut Microbiota." *Nature*, Macmillan Publishers Limited, 17 Sept. 2014, www.nature.com/nature/journal/v514/n7521/ful

2) l/nature13793.html.

3) Fowler, Sharon P.G., et al. "Diet Soda Intake Is Associated with Long-Term Increases in Waist Circumference in a Biethnic Cohort of Older Adults: The San Antonio Longitudinal Study of Aging." *Journal of the American Geriatrics Society*, Wiley Online Library, 17 Mar. 2015, onlinelibrary.wiley.com/wol1/doi/10.1111/jgs.13376/abstract.

4) Owen, Neville, et al. "Sedentary Behavior: Emerging Evidence for a New Health Risk." *Mayo Clinic Proceedings*, Mayo Foundation for Medical Education and Research, Dec. 2010, www.ncbi.nlm.nih.gov/pmc/articles/PMC2996155/.

CHAPTER 3: NUTRITIONAL INTAKE

1) "Differentiation of ALA (Plant Sources) from DHA + EPA (Marine Sources) as Dietary Omega-3 Fatty Acids for Human Health." *The Source for Objective Science-Based DHA/EPA Omega-3 Information*, DHA/EPA Omega-3 Institute, www.dhaomega3.org/Overview/ Differentiation-of-ALA-plant-sources-fro m-DHA-+-EPA-marine-sources-as-Dietary-Omega-3-Fatty-Acids-for-Human-Health.

2) Maroon, J C, and J W Bost. "Omega-3 Fatty Acids (Fish Oil) as an Anti-Inflammatory: an Alternative to Nonsteroidal Anti-Inflammatory Drugs for Discogenic Pain." *Surgical Neurology.*, U.S. National Library of Medicine, Apr. 2006, www.ncbi.nlm.nih. gov/pubmed/16531187.

3) Kohli, Payal, and Bruce D Levy. "Resolvins and Protectins: Mediating Solutions to Inflammation." *British Journal of Pharmacology*, Blackwell Publishing Ltd, Oct. 2009, www.ncbi.nlm. nih.gov/pmc/articles/PMC2785519/.

4) Talukdar, Saswata, et al. "GPR120 Is an Omega-3 Fatty Acid Receptor Mediating Potent Anti-Inflammatory and Insulin-Sensitizing Effects." *Cell*, Elsevier, 2 Sept. 2010, www.cell.com/ cell/fulltext/S0092-8674(10)00888-3.

5) Osher, Y, and R H Belmaker. "Omega-3 Fatty Acids in Depression: a Review of Three Studies." *CNS Neuroscience & Therapeutics.*, U.S. National Library of Medicine, 2009, www.ncbi.nlm.nih.gov/ pubmed/19499625.

6) Freeman, M. P., et al. "Omega-3 fatty acids: evidence basis for treatment and future research in psychiatry". *The Journal of clinical psychiatry*, U.S. National Library of Medicine, Dec. 2006, https:// www.ncbi.nlm.nih.gov/pubmed/17194275.

7) Richardson, A J. "Omega-3 Fatty Acids in ADHD and Related Neurodevelopmental Disorders." *International Review of Psychiatry (Abingdon, England).*, U.S. National Library of Medicine, Apr. 2006, www.ncbi.nlm.nih.gov/pubmed/16777670.

8) "Omega-3 Fatty Acids: An Essential Contribution". *The Nutrition Source*, Harvard School of Public Health, 26 May 2015, https://www.hsph.harvard.edu/nutritionsource/omega-3-fats/.

9) Undurraga, Dawn, et al. "Superbugs Invade American Supermarkets." *Meat and Antibiotics - 2013 Meat Eater's Guide | Meat Eater's Guide to Climate Change + Health | Environmental Working Group*, Environmental Working Group, www.ewg.org/meateatersguide/superbugs/.

10) Pariza, M W. "Perspective on the Safety and Effectiveness of Conjugated Linoleic Acid." *The American Journal of Clinical Nutrition.*, U.S. National Library of Medicine, June 2004, www.ncbi.nlm.nih.gov/pubmed/15159246.

11) Dhiman, T R, et al. "Conjugated Linoleic Acid Content of Milk from Cows Fed Different Diets."*Journal of Dairy Science.*, U.S. National Library of Medicine, Oct. 1999, www.ncbi.nlm.nih.gov/pubmed/10531600.

12) Ponnampalam, E N, et al. "Effect of Feeding Systems on Omega-3 Fatty Acids, Conjugated Linoleic Acid and Trans Fatty Acids in Australian Beef Cuts: Potential Impact on Human Health." *Asia Pacific Journal of Clinical Nutrition.*, U.S. National Library of Medicine, 2006, www.ncbi.nlm.nih.gov/pubmed/16500874.

13) Gunnars, Kris. "Grass-Fed vs Grain-Fed Beef — What's The Difference?" *Healthline*, Healthline Media, 8 Aug. 2013, www.healthline.com/nutrition/grass-fed-vs-grain-fed-beef.

14) Hebeisen, D F, et al. "Increased Concentrations of Omega-3 Fatty Acids in Milk and Platelet Rich Plasma of Grass-Fed Cows." *International Journal for Vitamin and Nutrition Research.*, U.S. National Library of Medicine, 1993, www.ncbi.nlm.nih.gov/pubmed/7905466.

15) Bonthuis, M, et al. "Dairy Consumption and Patterns of Mortality of Australian Adults." *Nature News*, Nature Publishing Group, 7 Apr. 2010, www.nature.com/ejcn/journal/v64/n6/abs/ejcn201045a.html.

16) Smit, Liesbeth A, and and Ana Baylin. "Liesbeth A Smit." *The American Journal of Clinical Nutrition*, American Society for Nutrition, 1 July 2010, ajcn.nutrition.org/content/92/1/34.

17) Warensjö, Eva, et al. "Stroke and Plasma Markers of Milk Fat Intake – a Prospective Nested Case-Control Study." *Nutrition Journal*, BioMed Central, 21 May 2009, nutritionj.biomedcentral. com/articles/10.1186/1475-2891-8-21.

18) Biong, A S, et al. "Intake of Milk Fat, Reflected in Adipose Tissue Fatty Acids and Risk of Myocardial Infarction: a Case I [Ndash] I Control Study." *Nature News*, Nature Publishing Group, 2 Nov. 2005, www. nature.com/ejcn/journal/v60/n2/full/1602307a.html.

19) Leech, Joe. "Vitamin K2: Everything You Need to Know." *Healthline*, Healthline Media, 4 June 2017, www.healthline.com/ nutrition/vitamin-k2.

20) Spronk, H M, et al. "Tissue-Specific Utilization of Menaquinone-4 Results in the Prevention of Arterial Calcification in Warfarin-Treated Rats." *Journal of Vascular Research.*, U.S. National Library of Medicine, 2003, www.ncbi.nlm.nih.gov/pubmed/14654717.

21) Shea, M. Kyla, and Rachel M. Holden. "Vitamin K Status and Vascular Calcification: Evidence from Observational and Clinical Studies." *Advances in Nutrition: An International Review Journal*, Advances in Nutrition, Mar. 2012, advances.nutrition.org/ content/3/2/158.full.pdf+html.

22) Pearson, Thomas A., et al. "Markers of Inflammation and Cardiovascular Disease: Application to Clinical and Public Health Practice: A Statement for Healthcare Professionals From the Centers for Disease Control and Prevention and the American Heart Association." *Circulation*, American Heart Association, Inc., 28 Jan. 2003, circ.ahajournals.org/content/107/3/499.full.

23) Tracy, Russell P. "Inflammation in Cardiovascular Disease: Cart, Horse, or Both?" *Circulation*, American Heart Association, Inc., 26 May 1998, circ.ahajournals.org/content/97/20/2000.full.

24) Szmitko, Paul E., et al. "New Markers of Inflammation and Endothelial Cell Activation: Part I." *Circulation*, American Heart Association, Inc., 21 Oct. 2003, circ.ahajournals.org/content/108/16/1917.long.

25) Säemann, M D, et al. "Anti-Inflammatory Effects of Sodium Butyrate on Human Monocytes: Potent Inhibition of IL-12 and up-Regulation of IL-10 Production." *FASEB Journal : Official Publication of the Federation of American Societies for Experimental Biology.*, U.S. National Library of Medicine, Dec. 2000, www.ncbi.nlm.nih.gov/pubmed/11024006.

26) Lührs, H, et al. "Butyrate Inhibits NF-KappaB Activation in Lamina Propria Macrophages of Patients with Ulcerative Colitis." *Scandinavian Journal of Gastroenterology.*, U.S. National Library of Medicine, Apr. 2002, www.ncbi.nlm.nih.gov/pubmed/11989838.

27) Hamer, H. M., et al. "Review Article: the Role of Butyrate on Colonic Function." *Alimentary Pharmacology & Amp Therapeutics*, Blackwell Publishing Ltd, 26 Oct. 2007, onlinelibrary.wiley.com/doi/10.1111/j.1365-2036.2007.03562.x/full.

28) Mama, Katie - Wellness. "Bone Broth Benefits and Uses | Wellness Mama." *Wellness Mama*, Wellness Mama, 6 Sept. 2016, wellnessmama.com/23777/bone-broth-benefits/.

29) Andersen, Charlotte H. "8 Reasons to Get In On the Bone Broth Trend." *Shape Magazine*, Meredith Corporation, 19 Oct. 2016, www.shape.com/healthy-eating/cooking-ideas/8-reasons-try-bone-broth.

30) Axe, Josh. "BoneBroth Benefits for Digestion, Arthritis, and Cellulite." *Dr. Axe*, Dr. Axe, 10 Oct. 2016, draxe.com/the-healing-power-of-bone-broth-for-digestion-arthritis-and-cellulite/.

31) Heid, Markham. "Does Bone Broth Really Have Health Benefits?" *Time*, Time, 6 Jan. 2016, time.com/4159156/bone-broth-health-benefits/.

32) "Paleo Foods: Bone Broth | Paleo Leap." *Paleo Leap | Paleo Diet Recipes & Tips*, Paleo Leap LLC, 5 July 2016, paleoleap.com/eat-this-bone-broth/.

33) "Bone Broth: What It Is, Why It's Good for You, and How to Make It." *Nourished Kitchen*, Nourished Kitchen, 8 May 2016, nourishedkitchen.com/bone-broth/.

CHAPTER 4: EXERCISE = LIFE EXTENSION

1) Harris, Carmen D., et al. "Adult Participation in Aerobic and Muscle-Strengthening Physical Activities - United States, 2011". *Centers for Disease Control and Prevention*, Centers for Disease Control and Prevention, 3 May 2013, https://www.cdc.gov/mmwr/preview/mmwrhtml/mm6217a2.htm?s_cid=m m6217a2_w.

2) Carek, P. J., S. E. Laibstain, and S. M. Carek. "Exercise for the treatment of depression and anxiety". *International journal of psychiatry in medicine*, U.S. National Library of Medicine, 2011, https://www.nc bi.nlm.nih.gov/pubmed/21495519.

3) Penhollow, Tina M., and Michael Young. "Sexual Desirability and Sexual Performance: Does Exercise and Fitness Really Matter?". *Electronic Journal of Human Sexuality*, University of Arkansas, 5 Oct. 2004, http://www.ejhs.org/volume7/fitness.html.

4) Gomez-Pinilla, Fernando, and Charles Hillman. "The Influence of Exercise on Cognitive Abilities". *Comprehensive Physiology*, U.S. National Library of Medicine, 13 Mar. 2014, https://www.ncbi.nlm.ni h.gov/pmc/articles/PMC3951958/.

5) Brinke, Lisanne F. Ten, et al. "Aerobic Exercise Increases Hippocampal Volume in Older Women with Probable Mild Cognitive Impairment: A 6-Month Randomized Controlled Trial". *British journal of sports medicine*, U.S. National Library of Medicine, 7 Apr. 2014, https://www.ncbi.nlm.nih.gov/pmc/articles/PM C4508129/.

6) Gatz, Margaret. "Educating the Brain to Avoid Dementia: Can Mental Exercise Prevent Alzheimer Disease?". *PLoS Medicine*, Public Library of Science, 25 Jan. 2005, https://www.ncbi.nlm.nih. gov/pm c/articles/PMC545200/.

7) Etgen, Thorleif, et al. "Physical Activity and Incident Cognitive Impairment in Elderly Persons". *Archives of Internal Medicine*, American Medical Association, 25 Jan. 2010, http://jamanetwork. com/journals/jama internalmedicine/fullarticle/774229.

8) Warburton, Darren E. R., Crystal Whitney Nicol, and Shannon S. D. Bredin. "Health benefits of physical activity: the evidence". *CMAJ: Canadian Medical Association Journal*, Canadian Medical Association, 14 Mar. 2006, https://www.ncbi.nlm.nih.gov/pmc/ articles/PMC1402378/.

9) Bernstein, L., B. E. Henderson, R. Hanisch, J. Sullivan-Halley, and R. K. Ross. "Physical exercise and reduced risk of breast cancer in young women". *Journal of the National Cancer Institute*, U.S. National Library of Medicine, 21 Sep. 1994, https://www.ncbi. nlm.nih.gov/pubmed/8072034.

10) Ballantyne, Coco. "Does Exercise Really Make You Healthier?". *Scientific American*, Nature America Inc., 2 Jan. 2009, https://www. scientificamerican.com/article/does-exercise-really-make/.

11) Brody, Jane E. "Even More Reasons to Get a Move On". *The New York Times*, The New York Times, 1 Mar. 2010, http://www. nytimes.com/2010/03/02/health/02brod.html.

12) Melov, Simon, Mark A. Tamopolsky, Kenneth Beckman, Krysta Felkey, and Alan Hubbard. "Resistance Exercise Reverses Aging in Human Skeletal Muscle". *PLoS ONE*, Public Library of Science, 23 May 2007, https://www.ncbi.nlm.nih.gov/pmc/ articles/PMC1866181/.

13) Safdar, Adeel, et al. "Endurance exercise rescues progeroid aging and induces systemic mitochondrial rejuvenation in mtDNA mutator mice". *Proceedings of the National Academy of Sciences of the*

United States of America, National Academy of Sciences, 8 Mar. 2011, https://www.ncbi.nlm.nih.gov/pmc/articles/PMC3053975/.

14) Diman, Aurelie, et al. "Nuclear respiratory factor 1 and endurance exercise promote human telomere transcription". *Science Advances*, American Association for the Advancement of Science, 1 Jul. 2016, http://advances.sciencemag.org/content/2/7/e16 00031.full.

CHAPTER 5: IN NEED OF SUPPLEMENTS?

1) "Antioxidants: In Depth". *National Center for Complementary and Integrative Health*, U.S. Department of Health and Human Services, 4 May 2016, https://nccih.nih.gov/health/antioxidants/introduction.htm.

2) Ristow, M. "Interview with Michael Ristow". *Aging*, U.S. National Library of Medicine, Jan. 2012, https://www.ncbi.nlm.nih.gov/pubmed/22317964.

3) Ristow, Michael, et al. "Antioxidants prevent health-promoting effects of physical exercise in humans". *Proceedings of the National Academy of Sciences*, National Acad Sciences, 31 Mar. 2009, http://www.pnas.org/content/106/21/8665.

4) Swanson, Jerry W. "This vitamin might lessen the severity of MS symptoms". *Mayo Clinic*, Mayo Foundation for Medical Education and Research, 4 Feb. 2016, https://www.mayoclinic.org/diseases-conditions/multiple-sclerosis/expert-answers/vitamin-d-and-ms/faq-20058258.

5) Children's Hospital & Research Center Oakland. "Casual link found between vitamin D, serotonin synthesis and autism in new study". *ScienceDaily*, ScienceDaily, 26 Feb. 2014, https://www.sciencedaily.com/releases/2014/02/140226110836.htm#.U2IoNnjAZBo.email.

6) Littlejohns, MSc Thomas J., et al. "Vitamin D and the risk of dementia and Alzheimer disease". *Neurology*, American Academy

of Neurology, 6 Aug. 2014, www.neurology.org/content/ early/2014/08/06/WNL.0000000000000755.short.

7) Osher, Y., and R. H. Belmaker. "Omega-3 fatty acids in depression: a review of three studies". *CNS neuroscience & therapeutics*, U.S. National Library of Medicine, 2009, https://www.ncbi.nlm. nih.gov/pubmed/19499625.

8) Freeman, M. P., et al. "Omega-3 fatty acids: evidence basis for treatment and future research in psychiatry". *The Journal of clinical psychiatry*, U.S. National Library of Medicine, Dec. 2006, https:// www.ncbi.nlm.nih.gov/pubmed/17194275.

9) Richardson, A. J. "Omega-3 fatty acids in ADHD and related neurodevelopmental disorders". *International review of psychiatry (Abingdon, England)*, U.S. National Library of Medicine, Apr. 2006, https://www.ncbi.nlm.nih.gov/pubmed/16777670.

10) "Omega-3 Fatty Acids: An Essential Contribution". *The Nutrition Source*, Harvard School of Public Health, 26 May 2015, https:// www.hsph.harvard.edu/nutritionsource/omega-3-fats/.

11) Kiecolt-Glaser, J. K., M. A. Belury, R. Andridge, W. B. Malarkey, and R. Glaser. "Omega-3 supplementation lowers inflammation and anxiety in medical students: a randomized controlled trial". *Brain, behavior, and immunity*, U.S. National Library of Medicine, Nov. 2011, https://www.ncbi.nlm.nih.go v/pubmed/21784145.

12) Li, K., T. Huang, J. Zheng, K. Wu, and D. Li. "Effect of marine-derived n-3 polyunsaturated fatty acids on C-reactive protein, interleukin 6 and tumor necrosis factor a: a meta-analysis". *PLoS ONE*, U.S. National Library of Medicine, 5 Feb. 2014, https://www.ncbi. nlm.nih.gov/pubmed/24505395.

13) Swanson, D., R. Block, and S. A. Mousa. "Omega-3 fatty acids EPA and DHA: health benefits throughout life". *Advances in nutrition (Bethesda, Md.)*, U.S. National Library of Medicine, Jan. 2012, https://www.ncbi.nlm.nih.gov/pubmed/22332096.

14) Simopoulos, A. P. "Omega-3 fatty acids in inflammation and autoimmune diseases". *Journal of the American College of Nutrition*, U.S.

National Library of Medicine, Dec. 2002, https://www.ncbi.nlm. nih.go v/pubmed/12480795.

15) Meagen, M., M. D. McCusker, M. Jane, and M. D. Grant-Kels. "Healing fats of the skin: the structural and immunologic roles of the w-6 and w-3 fatty acids". *Clinics in Dermatology*, Elsevier, 29 Jun. 2010, http://www.sciencedirect.com/science/article/pii/ S0738081X10000441.

16) Montgomery, P., J. R. Burton, R. P. Sewell, T. F. Spreckelsen, and A. J. Richardson. "Fatty acids and sleep in UK children: subjective and pilot objective sleep results from the DOLAB study -- a randomized controlled trial". *Journal of sleep research*, U.S. National Library of Medicine, Aug. 2014, https://www.ncbi.nlm.nih.gov/ pubmed/24605819.

17) Hansen, Anita L., et al. "Fish Consumption, Sleep, Daily Functioning, and Heart Rate Variability". *Journal of Clinical Sleep Medicine: JCSM: Official Publication of the American Academy of Sleep Medicine*, American Academy of Sleep Medicine, 15 May 2014, https://www.ncbi.nlm.nih.gov/pmc/articles/PMC4013386/.

18) Offman, Elliot, et al. "Steady-State Bioavailability of Prescription Omega-3 on a Low-Fat Diet Is Significantly Improved with a Free Fatty Acid Formulation Compared with an Ethyl Ester Formulation: the ECLIPSE II Study." Vascular Health and Risk Management, Dove Medical Press, 2013, www.ncbi.nlm.nih.gov/ pmc/articles/PMC3794864/.

19) Nishida, Yasuhiro, Eiji Yamashita, and Wataru Miki. "Quenching Activities of Common Hydrophilic and Lipophilic Antioxidants against Singlet Oxygen Using Chemiluminescence Detection System". *Carotenoid Science*, Institute for Food Science Research, Jun. 2001, http://www.bioastinturkiye.com/bilimsel_pdf/BioAstin-Astaxanthin-Antioksidan.pdf.

20) Kidd, P. "Astaxanthin, cell membrane nutrient with diverse clinical benefits and anti-aging potential". *Alternative medicine review:*

a journal of clinical therapeutic, U.S. National Library of Medicine, Dec. 2014, https://www.ncbi.nlm.nih.gov/pubmed/22214255.

21) Daniells, Stephen. "Astaxanthin may protect skin from within: Study". *nutraingredients-usa.com*, nutraingredients-usa.com, 13 Feb. 2017, http://www.nutraingredients-usa.com/Research/Astaxanth in-may-protect-skin-from-within-Study.

22) Camera, E., et al. "Astaxanthin, canthaxanthin and beta-carotene differently affect UVA-induced oxidative damage and expression of oxidative stress-responsive enzymes". *Experimental dermatology*, U.S. National Library of Medicine, 18 Sep. 2008, https://www. ncbi.nlm.nih.gov/pubmed/18803658.

23) Satoh, Akira, et al. "Preliminary Clinical Evaluation of Toxicity and Efficacy of A New Astaxanthin-rich *Haematococcus pluvialis* Extract". *Journal of Clinical Biochemistry and Nutrition*, The Society for Free Radical Research Japan, 25 Apr. 2009, https://www.ncbi. nlm.nih.gov/pmc/articles/PMC2675019/.

24) Mercola, Joseph. "Astaxanthin: Nature's Most Powerful Antioxidant". *Mercola.com*, Dr. Mercola's Natural Health News-letter, 10 Feb. 2013, https://articles.mercola.com/sites/articles/ archive/2013/02/10/cysewki-discloses-astaxanthin-benefits. aspx.

25) Axe, Josh. "Astaxanthin Benefits 6000x Stronger Than Vitamin C". *Dr. Axe*, Dr. Axe, 21 Jun. 2017, https://draxe.com/ astaxanthin-benefits/.

26) Proksch, E., et al. "Oral supplementation of specific collagen peptides has beneficial effects on human skin physiology: a double-blind, placebo-controlled study". *Skin pharmacology and physiology*, U.S. National Library of Medicine, 14 Aug. 2013, https://www. ncbi.nlm.nih.gov/pubmed/23949208.

27) Asserin, J., E. Lati, T. Shioya, and J. Prawitt. "The effect of oral collagen peptide supplementation on skin moisture and the dermal collagen network: evidence from an ex vivo model and randomized, placebo-controlled clinical trials". *Journal of cosmetic dermatology*,

U.S. National Library of Medicine, 12 Sep. 2015, https://www. ncbi.nlm.nih.gov/pubmed/26362110.

28) Sibilla, Sara, Martin Godfrey, Sarah Brewer, Anil Budh-Raja, and Licia Genovese. "An Overview of the Beneficial Effects of Hydrolysed Collagen as a Nutraceutical on Skin Properties: Scientific Background and Clinical Studies". *Open Access*, The Open Nutraceutical Journal, 2015, https://benthamopen.com/ contents/pdf/TONUTRAJ/TONUTRAJ-8-29.pdf.

29) Asserin, Jérome, et al. "The Effect of Oral Collagen Peptide Supplementation on Skin Moisture and the Dermal Collagen Network: Evidence from an Ex Vivo Model and Randomized, Placebo-Controlled Clinical Trials." *Journal of Cosmetic Dermatology*, John Wiley & Sons, 12 Sept. 2015, onlinelibrary. wiley.com/doi/10.1111/jocd.12174/full.

30) Frestedt, Joy L, et al. "A Whey-Protein Supplement Increases Fat Loss and Spares Lean Muscle in Obese Subjects: a Randomized Human Clinical Study." *Nutrition & Metabolism*, BioMed Central, 2008, www.ncbi.nlm.nih.gov/pmc/articles/PMC2289832/.

31) Bendtsen, Line Q., Janne K. Corenzen, Nathalie T. Bendsen, Charlotte Rasmusson, and Arne Astrup. "Effect of Dairy Proteins on Appetite, Energy Expenditure, Body Weight, and Composition: a Review of the Evidence from Controlled Clinical Trials". *Advances in Nutrition: An International Review Journal*, American Society for Nutrition, 1 Jul. 2013, http://advances.nutrition.org/ content/4/4/418.full

32) Annigan, Jan. "Does Whey Protein Help You Recover Faster?" *Healthy Eating | SF Gate*, SF Gate, healthyeating.sfgate.com/ whey-protein-recover-faster-7396.html.

33) Hayes, A, and P J Cribb. "Effect of Whey Protein Isolate on Strength, Body Composition and Muscle Hypertrophy during Resistance Training." *Current Opinion in Clinical Nutrition and Metabolic Care.*, U.S. National Library of Medicine, Jan. 2008, www.ncbi.nlm.nih.gov/pubmed/18090657.

34) "How to Boost Your Immune System." *Harvard Health*, Harvard Health Publishing, Sept. 2014, www.health.harvard.edu/staying-healthy/how-to-boost-your-immune-system.

35) Mangano, Kelsey M., et al. "Dietary Protein Is Beneficial to Bone Health under Conditions of Adequate Calcium Intake: an Update on Clinical Research." *Current Opinion in Clinical Nutrition and Metabolic Care*, U.S. National Library of Medicine, Jan. 2014, www.ncbi.nlm.nih.gov/pmc/articles/PMC4180248/.

36) Volek, Jeff S. "Creatine: The next Anti-Aging Supplement? - Nutrition Express Articles." *Nutrition Express*, HealthNotes, 2016, www.nutritionexpress.com/article+index/authors/jeff+s+volek+phd+rd/showarticle.aspx?id=907.

37) The Royal Society. "Boost Your Brain Power: Creatine, A Compound Found In Muscle Tissue, Found To Improve Working Memory And General Intelligence." *ScienceDaily*, ScienceDaily, 13 August 2003. https://www.sciencedaily.com/releases/2003/08/030813070944.htm.

38) Tarnopolsky, M A, and M F Beal. "Potential for Creatine and Other Therapies Targeting Cellular Energy Dysfunction in Neurological Disorders." *Annals of Neurology.*, U.S. National Library of Medicine, May 2001, www.ncbi.nlm.nih.gov/pubmed/11357946.

39) Rae, C, et al. "Oral Creatine Monohydrate Supplementation Improves Brain Performance: a Double-Blind, Placebo-Controlled, Cross-over Trial." *Proceedings. Biological Sciences.*, U.S. National Library of Medicine, 22 Oct. 2003, www.ncbi.nlm.nih.gov/pubmed/14561278.

40) Rawson, E S, and A C Venezia. "Use of Creatine in the Elderly and Evidence for Effects on Cognitive Function in Young and Old." *Amino Acids.*, U.S. National Library of Medicine, May 2011, www.ncbi.nlm.nih.gov/pubmed/21394604.

41) Mawer, Rudy. "10 Health and Performance Benefits of Creatine." *Healthline*, Healthline Media, 22 Apr. 2016, www.healthline.com/nutrition/10-benefits-of-creatine.

42) Benzi, G, and A Ceci. "Creatine as Nutritional Supplementation and Medicinal Product." *The Journal of Sports Medicine and Physical Fitness.*, U.S. National Library of Medicine, Mar. 2001, www.ncbi. nlm.nih.gov/pubmed/11317142.

43) Mawer, Rudy. "10 Health and Performance Benefits of Creatine." *Healthline*, Healthline Media, 22 Apr. 2016, www.healthline.com/ nutrition/10-benefits-of-creatine.

44) McMorris, T, et al. "Effect of Creatine Supplementation and Sleep Deprivation, with Mild Exercise, on Cognitive and Psychomotor Performance, Mood State, and Plasma Concentrations of Catecholamines and Cortisol." *Psychopharmacology.*, U.S. National Library of Medicine, Mar. 2006, www.ncbi.nlm.nih.gov/pubmed/ 16416332.

45) Jäger, Ralf, et al. "Analysis of the Efficacy, Safety, and Regulatory Status of Novel Forms of Creatine." *Amino Acids*, Springer Vienna, May 2011, www.ncbi.nlm.nih.gov/pmc/articles/PMC3080578/.

46) Galvan, Elfego, et al. "Acute and Chronic Safety and Efficacy of Dose Dependent Creatine Nitrate Supplementation and Exercise Performance." *Journal of the International Society of Sports Nutrition*, BioMed Central, 31 Mar. 2016, jissn.biomedcentral.com/ articles/10.1186/s12970-016-0124-0.

47) Voss, Gretchen. "The Risks of Anti-Aging Medicine." *CNN*, Cable News Network, 14 Dec. 2016, www.cnn.com/2011/12/28/health/ age-youth-treatment-medication/.

CHAPTER 6: INTERMITTENT FASTING

1) Martin, Bronwen, Mark P. Mattson, and Stuart Maudsley. "Caloric restriction and intermittent fasting: Two potential diets for successful brain aging". *Ageing research reviews*, U.S. National Library of Medicine, 8 Aug. 2006, https://www.ncbi.nlm.nih.gov/pmc/ articles/PMC2622429/.

2) Lee, J., W. Duan, J. M. Long, D. K. Ingram, and M. P. Mattson. "Dietary restriction increases the number of newly generated neural cells, and induces BDNF expression, in the dentate gyrus of rats". *Journal of Molecular Neuroscience: MN*, U.S. National Library of Medicine, Oct. 2000, https://www.ncbi.nlm.nih.gov/pubmed/11220789.

3) Mattson, M. P. "Energy intake, meal frequency, and health: a neurobiological perspective". *Annual review of nutrition*, U.S. National Library of Medicine, 2005, https://www.ncbi.nlm.nih.gov/pubmed/16011467.

4) Dean, Wenzhen, et al. "Dietary restriction normalizes glucose metabolism and BDNF levels, slows disease progression, and increases survival in huntingtin mutant mice". *Proceedings of the National Academy of Sciences of the United States of America*, The National Academy of Sciences, 4 Mar. 2003, https://www.ncbi.nlm.nih.gov/pmc/articles/PMC151440/.

5) Li, Liaoliao, Zhi Wang, and Zhiyi Zuo. "Chronic Intermittent Fasting Improves Cognitive Functions and Brain Structures in Mice". *PLoS ONE*, Public Library of Science, 3 Jun. 2013, http://journals.plos.org/plosone/article?id=10.1371/journal.pone.0066069.

6) Diniz, B. S., and A. L. Teixeira. "Brain-derived neurotrophic factor and Alzheimer's disease: physiopathology and beyond". *Neuromolecular medicine*, U.S. National Library of Medicine, Dec. 2011, https://www.ncbi.nlm.nih.gov/pubmed/21898045.

7) Lee, Bun-Hee, and Yong-Ku Kim. "The Roles of BDNF in the Pathophysiology of Major Depression and in Antidepressant Treatment". *Psychiatry Investigation*, Korean Neuropsychiatric Association, 23 Nov. 2010, https://www.ncbi.nlm.nih.gov/pmc/articles/PMC3022308/.

8) Beilharz, Jessica E., Jayanthi Maniam, and Margaret J. Morris. "Diet-Induced Cognitive Deficits: The Roles of Fat and Sugar, Potential Mechanisms and Nutritional Interventions". *Nutrients*,

MDPI, 12 Aug. 2015, https://www.ncbi.nlm.nih.gov/pmc/articles/ PMC4555146/.

9) Halagappa, V. K., et al. "Intermittent fasting and caloric restriction ameliorate age-related behavioral deficits in the triple-transgenic mouse model of Alzheimer's disease". *Neurobiology of disease*, U.S. National Library of Medicine, Apr. 2007, https://www.ncbi.nlm. nih.gov/pubmed/17306982.

10) Martin, Bronwen, Mark P. Mattson, and Stuart Maudsley. "Caloric restriction and intermittent fasting: Two potential diets for successful brain aging". *Ageing research reviews*, U.S. National Library of Medicine, 8 Aug. 2006, https://www.ncbi.nlm.nih.gov/pmc/ articles/PMC2622429/.

11) Duan, W., and M. P. Mattson. "Dietary restriction and 2-deoxy-glucose administration improve behavioral outcome and reduce degeneration of dopaminergic neurons in models of Parkinson's disease". *Journal of Neuroscience Research*, U.S. National Library of Medicine, 15 Jul. 1999, https://www.ncbi.nlm.nih.gov/ pubmed/10398297.

12) Arumugam, Thiruma V., et al. "Age and Energy Intake Interact to Modify Cell Stress Pathways and Stroke Outcome". *Annals of neurology*, U.S. National Library of Medicine, Jan. 2010, https://www. ncbi.nlm.nih.gov/pmc/articles/PMC2844782/.

13) Brandhorst, S., et al. "A Periodic Diet that Mimics Fasting Promotes Multi-System Regeneration, Enhanced Cognitive Performance, and Healthspan". *Cell metabolism*, U.S. National Library of Medicine, 7 Jul. 2015, https://www.ncbi.nlm.nih.gov/ pubmed/26094889.

14) Brandhorst, Sebastian, et al. "A Periodic Diet that Mimics Fasting Promotes Multi-System Regeneration, Enhanced Cognitive Performance, and Healthspan". *Cell Metabolism*, Elsevier Inc., 18 Jun. 2015, http://www.cell.com/cell-metabolism/fulltext/S1550-4131(15)00224-7.

15) Wei, Min, et al. "Life Span Extension by Calorie Restriction Depends on Rim15 and Transcription Factors Downstream of Ras/PKA, Tor, and Sch9". *PLoS Genetics*, Public Library of Science, 25 Jan. 2008, http://journals.plos.org/plosgenetics/article?id=10.1371/journal.pgen.0040013.

16) Fontana, Luigi, Linda Partridge, and Valter D. Longo. "Dietary Restriction, Growth Factors and Aging: from yeast to humans". *Science (New York, N.Y.)*, U.S. National Library of Medicine, 16 Apr. 2010, https://www.ncbi.nlm.nih.gov/pmc/articles/PMC3607354/.

17) Lee, C., et al. "Fasting cycles retard growth of tumors and sensitize a range of cancer cell types to chemotherapy". *Science translational medicine*, U.S. National Library of Medicine, 7 Mar. 2012, https://www.ncbi.nlm.nih.gov/pubmed/22323820.

18) Safdie, F. M., et al. "Fasting and cancer treatment in humans: A case series report". *Aging*, U.S. National Library of Medicine, 31 Dec. 2009, https://www.ncbi.nlm.nih.gov/pubmed/20157582/.

19) Brandhorst, Sebastian, et al. "A Periodic Diet that Mimics Fasting Promotes Multi-System Regeneration, Enhanced Cognitive Performance, and Healthspan". *Cell Metabolism*, Elsevier Inc., 18 Jun. 2015, http://www.cell.com/cell-metabolism/fulltext/S1550-4131(15)00224-7.

20) Block, Melissa. "Discovering The Genetic Controls That Dictate Life Span". *Print Friendly*, LifeExtension, Jun. 2002, http://www.lifeextension.com/Magazine/2002/6/report_kenyon/Page-01?p=1.

21) Horne, Benjamin D., Joseph B. Muhlestein, and Jeffrey L. Anderson. "Health effects of intermittent fasting: hormesis or harm? A systematic review". *Nutrition*, American Society for Nutrition, 1 Jul. 2015, http://ajcn.nutrition.org/content/early/2015/07/01/ajcn.115.109553.full.pdf.

22) Ho, K. Y., et al. "Fasting enhances growth hormone secretion and amplifies the complex rhythms of growth hormone secretion in

man". *Journal of Clinical Investigation*, U.S. National Library of Medicine, Apr. 1988, https://www.ncbi.nlm.nih.gov/pmc/articles/PMC329619/.

23) Hartman, M. L., et al. "Augmented growth hormone (GH) secretory burst frequency and amplitude mediate enhanced GH secretion during a two-day fast in normal men". *The journal of clinical endocrinology and metabolism*, U.S. National Library of Medicine, Apr. 1992, https://www.ncbi.nlm.nih.gov/pubmed/1548337.

24) Lanzi, R., et al. "Elevated insulin levels contribute to the reduced growth hormone (GH) response to GH-releasing hormone in obese subjects". *Metabolism: clinical and experimental*, U.S. National Library of Medicine, Sep. 1999, https://www.ncbi.nlm.nih.gov/pubmed/10484056.

25) Ji, Shaonin, Ran Guan, Stuart J. Frank, and Joseph L. Messina. "Insulin Inhibits Growth Hormone Signaling via the Growth Hormone Receptor/JAK2/STAT5B Pathway". *Journal of Biological Chemistry*, American Society for Biochemistry and Molecular Biology, 7 May 1999, http://www.jbc.org/content/274/19/13434.abstract.

26) Heilbronn, L. K., S. R. Smith, C. K. Martin, S. D. Anton, and E. Ravussin. "Alternate-day fasting in nonobese subjects: effects on body weight, body composition, and energy metabolism". *The American Journal of Clinical Nutrition*, U.S. National Library of Medicine, Jan. 2005, https://www.ncbi.nlm.nih.gov/pubmed/15640462.

27) Mansell, P. I., I. W. Fellows, and I. A. Macdonald. "Enhanced thermogenic response to epinephrine after 48-h starvation in humans". *The American Journal of Physiology*, U.S. National Library of Medicine, Jan. 1990, https://www.ncbi.nlm.nih.gov/pubmed/2405717.

28) Zauner, C., et al. "Resting energy expenditure in short-term starvation is increased as a result of an increase in serum

norepinephrine". *The American Journal of Clinical Nutrition*, U.S. National Library of Medicine, Jun. 2000, https://www.ncbi.nlm. nih.gov/pubmed/10837292.

29) Barnosky, Adrienne R., Kristin K. Hoddy, Terry G. Unterman, and Krista A. Varady. "Intermittent fasting vs daily calorie restriction for type 2 diabetes prevention: a review of human findings". *Translational Research*, Mosby, 12 Jun. 2014, http://www. sciencedirect.com/science/article/pii/S193152441400200X.

30) Barnosky, Adrienne R., Kristin K. Hoddy, Terry G. Unterman, and Krista A. Varady. "Intermittent fasting vs daily calorie restriction for type 2 diabetes prevention: a review of human findings". *Translational Research*, Mosby, 12 Jun. 2014, http://www. sciencedirect.com/science/article/pii/S193152441400200X.

31) Johnson, J. B., et al. "Alternate day calorie restriction improves clinical findings and reduces markers of oxidative stress and inflammation in overweight adults with moderate asthma". *Free radical biology & medicine*, U.S. National Library of Medicine, 1 Mar. 2007, https://www.ncbi.nlm.nih.gov/pubmed/17291990/.

32) Aksungar, F. B., A. E. Topkaya, and M. Akyildiz. "Interleukin-6, C-reactive protein and biochemical parameters during prolonged intermittent fasting". *Annals of nutrition & metabolism*, U.S. National Library of Medicine, 2007, https://www.ncbi.nlm.nih. gov/pubmed/17374948.

33) Johnson, J. B., et al. "Alternate day calorie restriction improves clinical findings and reduces markers of oxidative stress and inflammation in overweight adults with moderate asthma". *Free radical biology & medicine*, U.S. National Library of Medicine, 1 Mar. 2007, https://www.ncbi.nlm.nih.gov/pubmed/17291990/.

34) Alirezaei, Mehrdad, et al. "Short-term fasting induces profound neuronal autophagy". *Autophagy*, Landes Bioscience, 16 Aug. 2010, https://www.ncbi.nlm.nih.gov/pmc/articles/PMC3106288/.

CHAPTER 7: WEIGHT LOSS

1) Deans, Emily. "Your Brain on Ketones". *Psychology Today*, Sussex Publishers, 18 Apr. 2011, https://www.psychologytoday.com/blog/ evolutionary-psychiatry/201104/your-brain-ketones.

CHAPTER 8: HEALTHY GUT-HEALTHY BRAIN

1) "Elaine Hsiao Lab". *Elaine Hsiao Lab at Caltech*, Caltech, http:// poo.caltech.edu/

2) Hsiao, Elaine Y. "Emerging Roles for the Gut Microbiome in Autism Spectrum Disorder."Biological Psychiatry, Society of Biological Psychiatry, 27 Aug. 2016, www.biologicalpsychiatryjournal.com/ article/S0006-3223(16)32724-X/fulltext.

3) Tito, Raul Y, et al. "Insights from Characterizing Extinct Human Gut Microbiomes". *PLOSone* (originally University of Oklahoma), College of Arts and Sciences, 12 Dec. 2012, http://journals.plos.org/plosone/article?id=10.1371/journal. pone.0051146.

4) Brown, Kirsty, et al. "Diet-Induced Dysbiosis of the Intestinal Microbiota and the Effects on Immunity and Disease". *Nutrients*, Multidisciplinary Digital Publishing Institute, 21 Aug. 2012, https://www.ncbi.nlm.nih.gov/pmc/articles/PMC3448089/.

5) Dantzer, Robert, et al. "From inflammation to sickness and depression: when the immune system subjugates the brain". *HHS Public Access*, U.S. National Library of Medicine, 10 Aug. 2010, https:// www.ncbi.nlm.nih.gov/pmc/articles/PMC2919277/.

6) Suez, Jotham, et al. "Artificial sweeteners induce glucose intolerance by altering the gut microbiota". *Nature*, Nature Publishing Group, 17 Sep. 2014, http://www.nature.com/nature/journal/ v514/n7521/full/nature13793.html?foxtrotcallback=true.

7) Zhang, Chenhong, et al. "Structural modulation of gut microbiota in life-long calorie-restricted mice". *Nature Communications*,

Nature Publishing Group, 16 July 2013, https://www.ncbi.nlm. nih.gov/pmc/articles/PMC3717500/.

8) Young, Emma. "Gut instincts: The secrets of your second brain". *NeuroscienceStuff*, 18 Dec. 2012, http://neuro sciencestuff.tumblr.com/post/38271759345/gut-instincts-the-secrets-of-your-second-brain.

9) Tillisch, Kirsten, et al. "Consumption of Fermented Milk Product With Probiotic Modulates Brain Activity". *HHS Public Access*, Elsevier Inc., 6 Mar. 2013, https://www.ncbi.nlm.nih.gov/pmc/ articles/PMC3839572/.

CHAPTER 9: SLEEP

1) Centers for Disease Control. "Insufficient Sleep Is a Public Health Problem". *Centers for Disease*

2) *Control and Prevention*, Centers for Disease Control and Prevention, 3 Sep. 2015, https://www.cdc.gov

3) /features/dssleep/.

4) Centers for Disease Control. "1 in 3 adults don't get enough sleep". *Centers for Disease Control and*

5) *Prevention*, Centers for Disease Control and Prevention, 16 Feb. 2016, https://www.cdc.gov/media/releases/2016/p0215-enough-sleep.html.

6) Van, H. P., G. Maislin, J. M. Mullington, and D. F. Dinges. "The cumulative cost of additional wakefulness: dose-response effects on neurobehavioral functions and sleep physiology from chronic sleep restriction and total sleep deprivation". *Sleep*, U.S. National Library of Medicine, 15 Mar. 2003, https://www.ncbi.nlm.nih.gov/ pubmed/12683469?dopt=Abstract.

7) Patel, Sanjay R., and Frank B. Hu. "Short sleep duration and weight gain: a systematic review".

8) *Obesity (Silver Spring, Md.)*, U.S. National Library of Medicine, 17 Jan. 2008, https://www.ncbi.nlm.ni h.gov/pmc/articles/PMC2723045/.

9) Knutson, Kristen L., and Eve Van Cauter. "Associations between sleep loss and increased risk of obesity and diabetes". *Annals of the New York Academy of Sciences*, U.S. National Library of Medicine, May 2008, https://www.ncbi.nlm.nih.gov/pmc/articles/PMC4394987/.

10) Ruesten, Anne Von, Cornelia Weikert, Ingo Fietze, and Heiner Boeing. "Association of Sleep Duration with Chronic Diseases in the European Prospective Investigation into Cancer and Nutrition (EPIC)-Potsdam Study". *PLoS ONE*, Public Library of Science, 25 Jan. 2012, https://www.ncbi.nlm.nih.gov/pmc/articles/PMC3266295/.

11) Drake, C., T. Roehrs, J. Shambroom, and T. Roth. "Caffeine effects on sleep taken 0, 3, or 6 hoursbefore going to bed". *Journal of clinical sleep medicine: JCSM: official publication of the American*

12) *Academy of Sleep Medicine*, U.S. National Library of Medicine, 15 Nov. 2013, https://www.ncbi.nlm.nih.gov/pubmed/24235903.

CHAPTER 10: YOUR BEST SKIN

1) Cui, Hang, et al. "Oxidative Stress, Mitochondrial Dysfunction, and Aging". *Journal of Signal Transduction*, Hindawi Publishing Corporation, 2012, www.ncbi.nlm.nih.gov/pmc/articles/PMC3184498/.

2) López-Armada, M J, et al. "Mitochondrial dysfunction and the inflammatory response". *Mitochondrion*, U.S. National Library of Medicine, Mar. 2013, www.ncbi.nlm.nih.gov/pubmed/23333405.

3) Danby, F W. "Nutrition and aging skin: sugar and glycation". *Clinics in dermatology*, U.S. National Library of Medicine, 2010, www.ncbi.nlm.nih.gov/pubmed/20620757.

4) Lobo, V., et al. "Free radicals, antioxidants and functional foods: Impact on human health". *Pharmacognosy Reviews*, Medknow Publications & Media Pvt Ltd, 2010, www.ncbi.nlm.nih.gov/pmc/articles/PMC3249911/.

5) Gkogkolou, Paraskevi, and Markus Böhm. "Advanced glycation end products: Key players in skin aging?". *Dermato-Endocrinology*, Landes Bioscience, 1 July 2012, www.ncbi.nlm.nih.gov/pmc/articles/PMC3583887/.

6) Safdar, Adeel, et al. "Endurance exercise rescues progeroid aging and induces systemic mitochondrial rejuvenation in mtDNA mutator mice". *Proceedings of the National Academy of Sciences of the United States of America*, National Academy of Sciences, 8 Mar. 2011, www.ncbi.nlm.nih.gov/pmc/articles/PMC3053975/.

7) Crane, Justin D, et al. "Exercise-Stimulated interleukin-15 is controlled by AMPK and regulates skin metabolism and aging". *Aging Cell*, John Wiley & Sons, Ltd, Aug. 2015, www.ncbi.nlm.nih.gov/pmc/articles/PMC4531076/.

8) Reynolds, Gretchen. "Younger Skin Through Exercise". *The New York Times*, The New York Times, 16 Apr. 2014, well.blogs.nytimes.com/2014/04/16/younger-skin-through-exercise/?_r=0.

CHAPTER 11: CONNECTION = HAPPINESS AND LONGEVITY?

1) Mineo, Liz. "Good genes are nice, but joy is better". *Harvard Gazette*, Harvard University, 11 Apr.

2) 2017, https://news.harvard.edu/gazette/story/2017/04/over-nearly-80-years-harvard-study-has-been-showing-how-to-live-a-healthy-and-happy-life/.

3) Waldinger, Robert J. and Marc S. Schulz. "What's Love Got To Do With It?: Social Functioning, Perceived Health, and Daily Happiness in Married Octogenarians". *HHS Public Access*, Psychol Aging, Jun. 2010, https://www.ncbi.nlm.nih.gov/pmc/articles/PMC2896234/.

4) "Harvard Study of Adult Development". *Harvard Second Generation Study*, Harvard, http://www.adultdevelopmentstudy.org/

83327642R00124

Made in the USA
Middletown, DE
10 August 2018